Routledge Revivals

The Psychology of Pierre Janet

Pierre Janet (1859 – 1947) is considered to be one of the founders of psychology, and pioneered research in the disciplines of psychology, philosophy and psychotherapy. Janet's most crucial research, particularly in the subjects of 'dissociation' and 'subconscious' - terms coined by him - is explored in this book, first published in 1952. As Janet did not publish much in English, these notes provide guidance on such areas of study as hysteria and hypnosis, obsessive thinking and the psychology of adaption. Elton Mayo's comprehensive collection is an important guide for any student with an interest in the history of psychology, psychopathology and social study, and Janet's revolutionary work in the field.

The Psychology of Pierre Janet

Elton Mayo

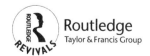

Routledge
Taylor & Francis Group

First published in 1952
by Routledge & Kegan Paul Ltd

This edition first published in 2013 by Routledge
2 Park Square, Milton Park, Abingdon, Oxon, OX14 4RN

Simultaneously published in the USA and Canada
by Routledge
711 Third Avenue, New York, NY 10017

Routledge is an imprint of the Taylor & Francis Group, an informa business

Publisher's Note
The publisher has gone to great lengths to ensure the quality of this reprint but
points out that some imperfections in the original copies may be apparent.

Disclaimer
The publisher has made every effort to trace copyright holders and welcomes
correspondence from those they have been unable to contact.

A Library of Congress record exists under LC control number: 52004812

ISBN 13: 978-0-415-73022-8 (hbk)
ISBN 13: 978-1-315-85046-7 (ebk)

THE PSYCHOLOGY OF
PIERRE JANET

BY
ELTON MAYO

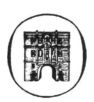

ROUTLEDGE & KEGAN PAUL LTD
BROADWAY HOUSE: CARTER LANE
LONDON, E.C.4

FIRST PUBLISHED IN ENGLAND

PRINTED IN GREAT BRITAIN BY
LUND HUMPHRIES
LONDON · BRADFORD

To

PIERRE JANET

1859-1947

In July, 1939, in the intervals of a conference in Paris, Janet expressed to me his complete conversion to the view that his observations could well be applied to the better understanding of social and industrial situations. For many years he had been doubtful on the point; but he gave evidence of his belief in the validity of our attempt by himself undertaking a similar study of the inmates of a prison in Paris. We had hoped for a period of more active collaboration, but, alas, the war put an end to these hopes in September, 1939. He survived the hardships of the war and read *The Social Problems of an Industrial Civilization*: I had a few words of acknowledgment from him expressing continued interest. I had hoped to have the benefit of his comment on these scanty notes.

E. M.

PREFACE

These notes on the work of Pierre Janet are merely *notes* and are not an adequate account of the many years of patient toil that Janet gave to clinical study. Since few, if any, of his more important works have been translated into English, this book is intended to provide some guidance for those who wish to read Janet in the original French as an aid to their studies of society or of industry. The book is not intended for medical students or for those who have a special interest in the problems of psychiatry. These notes were originally written for a few colleagues whose work demanded close attention to the difficult social, personal, and administrative problems of our time. In study of the particular situation — not any generalized problem of the textbooks — Janet's guidance has been found by them most useful. And it is at the instance of my colleagues that I publish the notes, despite their obvious insufficiency.

I should like to express my deepest gratitude to my secretary, Mrs. Selena Gardner, for her patient care in preparing the manuscript and proofs and to Miss Margaret C. Williams for the index.

E. M.

Graduate School of Business Administration
Harvard University
May 22, 1947

CONTENTS

THE PSYCHOLOGY OF
PIERRE JANET

I

PSYCHOPATHOLOGY
AND SOCIAL STUDY

Jerome K. Jerome, a writer who in these days is *démodé* and unread, tells somewhere of an idle afternoon he spent in the British Museum reading a large book that happened to his hand—a medical encyclopedia. In the course of some agitated hours thus spent, he discovered that he suffered from every ailment known to man with the sole exception of "housemaid's knee." I have sometimes thought that this is the general effect upon many members of many audiences that listen in these days to well-intended lectures on mental hygiene. The more intelligent and sensitive come gradually to believe that they detect in themselves symptoms of hysteria, obsession, schizophrenia, and paranoia; and they hear the concluding lectures in alarmed silence. The less intelligent or less sensitive members of the audience, on the other hand, tend to detect these same symptoms in all their friends and, finally, in the lecturer himself. Sometimes they become a little difficult socially. Evidently there is something in the topic

—mental hygiene—which makes it far from easy to present clearly and intelligently. I shall begin accordingly by giving some attention to the question as to what this difficulty is.

The difficulty is not simple but manifold. In the first place, the audience is not directly familiar with the facts: few people are intimately acquainted with even such apparently minor variations from the ordinary as hysteria, hypnosis, obsessive anxiety, or the characteristic phenomena of compulsion. If we hark back for a moment to William James's distinction between *knowledge-of-acquaintance* (direct familiarity) and *knowledge-about* (logical insight), we may fairly claim that where direct familiarity is at a minimum the development of any considerable insight is improbable or impossible. Consequently the lecturer is faced with the difficult task of attempting to communicate descriptive knowledge and logical insight simultaneously—an attempt which may result in considerable confusion not only for the audience but in the lectures themselves.

Nor is this all. The lecturer is frequently a clinician of considerable experience and consequently realizes clearly the great gulf that is fixed between the scientific abstractions of the laboratory and the actual complexity of the clinical situation.

In any developed science there is, of necessity, a wide gap between the diverse facts of observation and those few types of observed fact which form the basis of important generalizations and from which a body of theory is then derived. For the very act of reducing observation to order involves the neglect of many pertinent facts; a theory which attempted to take account of everything would be smothered by its own complexity. Thus all generalizations and theories necessarily refer to artificially simplified situations.[1]

The study of medicine is perhaps the only form of education which clearly and explicitly instructs the student to change his method and his conception of method as he walks out of the laboratory and into the hospital clinic. In the laboratory, simple assumptions and highly elaborated logic; in the clinic, complicated fact and simple logic. The clinician therefore has been trained to patient observation, to suspicion of brilliant flights of reasoning, and to a wary alertness for unexpected developments. It is inevitable that he should attempt, and rightly, to inculcate just such a point of view. Excellent as this procedure is, it does not make for that ease of communication which characterizes the demonstration of a complex logic—a complexity that is systematically patterned.

Finally, another difficulty: it is customary for lectures on mental hygiene to include, more or less, the whole psychiatric field. Neurological lesions and pathology, the major psychoses, the psychoneuroses—all these, as well as more ordinary maladjustments, come in for attention. And this is the last fatal complication—fatal, that is, for general understanding. So immense a descriptive load cannot be mentally

---

[1] T. North Whitehead, "Social Motives in Economic Activities," *Occupational Psychology*, vol. XII, no. 4 (Autumn, 1938), p. 171.

carried by those who have no direct acquaintance with such situations.

At the very beginning of this book I am therefore faced with a need to avoid or at least minimize these difficulties. I propose accordingly to confine my attention, so far as may be, to what Freud has called the psychopathology of everyday life. But in doing this I shall not fling my net so wide as Freud; for the most part I shall be considering the problem of obsessive thinking. My justification in this is twofold: First, it is in this area that modern psychopathology has made its most certain and completest contribution—it might, indeed, be said that the problem is clinically, if not practically, solved. And, second, I shall have an additional advantage in that every one of us who has the remotest claim to intelligence has at one time or other experienced something of obsessive disability. At one sweep, therefore, we may banish the disadvantages of unfamiliarity that I have indicated; for I shall be discussing the problems of the office, the street, and the home. Obsessive thinking is the inevitable variation from the norm that upon occasion afflicts you—and me. I shall, of course, need to give close attention to the work of Janet and others. I shall even be compelled for a time to follow somewhat intricate investigations of hysteria, for Janet begins by studying hysteria and is thus led to observe obsessive states and to distinguish them sharply from hysterical attacks. It is true that hysteria has small personal interest of a direct kind for most of us, whereas obsession is closely akin to many of our passing moods. But to understand the significance for us and for our society of these modern inquiries, we must understand where and how these modern researches began.

First of all, however, a word in passing as to what we mean by sanity. This is not a question of logical or verbal definition; on the contrary, it is a question of description. What are the situations to which ordinarily we apply the term "sane" as a descriptive epithet? Obviously, to any situation in which an individual clearly comprehends the activities of other persons about him, and relates himself to such activities by responsive speech and action in a manner that is satisfactory to the group and to himself. This description is no more than a first rough approximation; a philosopher might ask questions as to different levels of relationship, different degrees of sanity. Such questions are important and will demand consideration later, but certain simpler matters demand our primary attention.

The first of these is the obvious comment that sanity is in part achievement. We tend commonly to think of sanity as wholly a natural endowment. While natural endowment is an important, perhaps the most important factor, it is also evident that the sanity of adulthood develops step by step from a happy infancy and adolescence to an undamaged maturity. The conditions, broadly speaking, therefore, are a good biological endowment, intelligent parents, and a

B

well-ordered community life to effect the necessary
social training. We little realize, those of us who have
been fortunate enough to approximate these conditions
in early life, how far-reaching these influences are.
The achievement is not merely what we ordinarily
term mental, it is also to an astonishing degree an
achieved conditioning of actual organic process.
Many years ago, and in a country remote from this,
I happened across a small home into which were
brought illegitimate children and their mothers.
Some children had been much neglected, outcasts
and without the society of their kind. These
children not only would snarl and spit like
wildcats on the approach of a stranger, they were
also characterized by a complete uncontrol of
the ordinary processes of defecation and micturition.
Textbooks in anatomy speak of such controls as auto-
nomic, a function of the vegetative nervous system.
One does not ordinarily realize the extent to which
social convention defies the anatomists and insists
upon the establishment of a degree of conditioned
control.

The works of Freud and Janet show that in the
majority of instances, and indeed typically, obsession
is the consequence of some grave defect in this conditioning and training—primarily social but, as Freud
has shown, possibly organic also. If it were not so,
the radical re-training undertaken by psychoanalysis
would be useless. This assertion anticipates the detailed consideration I shall give the work of an

eminent clinician. But I make the assertion in order
that I may begin at once by giving certain simple
instances within my own experience. Almost forty
years ago in London I did some voluntary work
in an institution known as the Working Men's College, then situated in Great Ormond Street. Founded
by Frederick Denison Maurice and others, this college was supposed to bring opportunities of cultural
development to working men in their evenings. It
was surprisingly successful, and an interesting experience for a young man. One evening, at supper, one
of the college chess players seated next to me suddenly turned and said with the utmost vicious empha-
sis that he was an atheist. He did not merely say it,
he clenched his teeth, scowled, and closed his fists.
Being young, I did not make the appropriate Victor-
ian response—I laughed at the dramatic overemphasis.
This evidently surprised him; extensive reading of
Ingersoll and McCabe had prepared him for sustained
pseudological controversy but not for laughter. He
began to justify himself, and I suddenly realized that
he was telling me how bitterly he detested the rector
of his parish and that this was the clue to his "atheism." He had fallen in love with and married a girl
who was Roman Catholic. The rector had refused
to marry them and in doing so had increased the
difficulty of their social situation. The man re-
sponded by becoming an "atheist," since this expedi-
ent was more likely than any other to distress the
rector. As I came to know him better I often heard

him in long and complicated controversy on religion, apparently adept in all the literature of the Rationalist Press Association. After one such discussion, I said to him, "You are not really an atheist, you merely hate your rector." He hesitated a moment, then said, "I was thinking of becoming a Roman Catholic." But this was almost confidential.

The comment I wish to make on this case is that an ordinary encounter with this individual would have led one to suppose that the logic of the literature he had read had converted him from his Episcopalian faith to "atheism." This indeed was his claim in conversation. Actually, it became clear that he had become an atheist before reading the writers of the Rationalist Press. The rector's action had disrupted his relation with his group, and the atheism was of the nature of an angry objection to the disruption. I do not know the end of the story, but evidently the disruption had driven him into new social associations, the college and his wife's coreligionists. I have no doubt that if these associations proved satisfactory the interest in rationalist literature dwindled to nothing. This species of passing obsession I shall again discuss in a later chapter.

Some years after this I was one of the university members of a joint committee appointed by an Australian university to organize the classwork of a local branch of the Workers' Educational Association. In this capacity I frequently had occasion to speak before meetings of various trade unions to ask their support of the movement to extend the opportunities of adult education. This support was usually freely accorded, but not without vigorous discussion, in which the university representatives were accused of bourgeois sympathy and prejudice. To some extent this was a species of game played by trade union members: it was a test of the university man to see if he could stand up to rough heckling and give as good as he got. If he could do this he earned chuckles of approval and the consent of the meeting; sometimes indeed they would vigorously applaud a telling point made against one of their own speakers.

But this was not true of all the union members. The back rows of seats at these meetings were haunted by men of a very different type—the representatives of the extreme, irreconcilable Left. These members had no sense of humor or of toleration; and we soon came to know that six of these men were the nucleus of the most savage and unrelenting opposition. In the course of years I came to know these six quite well. When I first knew them, the extreme party called itself Socialist, and the six were the leaders of the local Socialist group. In the years that followed, the extreme party became the I.W.W., then Bolshevist, then Communist. No matter what the change of name or nominal change of doctrine, it was always the same six that led at union meetings, spoke from soap boxes in the public parks, and organized opposition to the university and all its works. The fact that I came to know them personally, and was even asked to supper in the leader's house, made no difference in their platform attitude to me and to what I was supposed to represent. But on other occasions they would talk freely to me in private and seemed to like to do so.

This curious relation between us enabled me to record the following observations:

1. These men had no friends except at the propagandist level. They seemed to be incapable of developing any kind of easy or automatic relationship with others. On the contrary, the need to achieve such relation was to them an emergency leading to crisis and energetic effort. Ordinary human relationship was impossible.

2. They had no capacity for conversation: at no time did I ever hear one try to amuse or to tell a story. In talking with me they alternated between silence, self-history, and oratory, which merely reproduced the sounding periods of their public utterances. They had one topic only, the compelling topic—the destruction of society.

3. All action was regarded as emergency action. It was completely impossible for them even to think about reform. At public meetings, indeed, nothing infuriated them so greatly as suggestions of reform. Revolution and de-

struction were the only possible meanings of action for them.

4. They regarded the world as a hostile place. Every belief and action implied that society existed not to give, but to deny, them opportunity. Furthermore, they believed this hostility to be active, not passive; they regarded everyone, even their immediate associates, as suspect of this conspiracy. In consequence of this, they did not easily collaborate even with each other. I once heard one of the six begin a speech in the Brisbane Domain with the sentence, "I am opposed to kings, capitalists, labor politicians, and trade union secretaries."

5. Everything they attempted was undertaken with immense and unreasoned "drive." Here again, however, any idea of routine collaboration or the "ordinary" was conspicuously absent. Every situation was conceived as emergency, crisis, drive. In spite of this, they always had a strong sense of impending calamity. The more strongly they drove for success, the privately certain they were of failure.

Five of the six were persons of considerable ability. Two, I believe, possessed conspicuous ability, and in happier circumstances might have been effective leaders. But their intelligent capacity actually served no purpose; they were, and remained, intellectual destroyers without any mitigation. For them, revolution meant the complete and utter destruction of society and nothing more. Although in conversation some admitted this, they at once added that they *wanted* to destroy society. It was evident that they had given no thought of what might lie beyond destruction.

So far, these observations have been generally descriptive. It happened that, after some time, one member of the group consulted a medical colleague who was my collaborator in the study of human adaptation. It was indeed knowledge of his participation that led to the consultation. The patient proved to have been an artisan, highly skilled, who rarely kept a job because he was unable to "take an order" from a boss or foreman. If anything said to him savored of command, he would instantly leave work with a comment to the effect that he was not going to be "ordered about." This was the individual who had begun the Domain speech by opposing himself equally to labor leaders, kings, and capitalists. Inquiry showed that he had been the only child in a family with a drunken and brutal father. It was the father's habit to come home drunk, beat his wife and child, and throw them into the street, after which he would lock the door and sleep off the effects of his bout. The man's recollections were of an infant's frightened night-wanderings in the streets with a terrified and unhappy mother. Commands in afterlife roused in him an attitude inspired by his father. After spending some time in medical care, the patient developed understanding of his personal situation and history and of the relation of his history to his difficulties of association with others. He developed a strong affection for his medical adviser and, under tutelage, a capacity for casual[2] friendships with other people. He made a good recovery. While he was in hospital, his political views were never once discussed, always his personal situation and personal history. When he left the hospital, it was discovered that he had completely lost interest in ideas of political revolution. He abandoned his former associates, took a clerical job and kept it.

The effect of this, to us extraordinary, case was to make us alert to the possible significance of the personal history of the other "destroyers." We did not succeed in establishing an intimacy sufficient to reproduce so dramatic a consequence with the other five. We were nevertheless able to extend somewhat, and to confirm, our original observations. For example, we found that the lack of ordinary friendships was not a late development but had characterized every stage of the personal history. At no time had any of these individuals achieved an easy intimate relationship of a routine character with others of their own generation. Many of them, unlike the artisan, had apparently had satisfactory or excellent parents; but there had been *no equivalent relationship with their own generation* outside the family. From this

---

[2]This is an important criterion.

curious situation they seemed to have derived a feeling of unadmitted superiority, which operated against their own age group; a resentment that they did not "belong"; an extravagant desire for leadership. The inevitable translation of every human encounter into emergency and crisis seemed to be related to this "outcast" conviction. This feeling of emergency was the characteristic personal attitude to others. The lack of capacity for conversation reflected the almost complete inexperience of routine and casual human associations. The oratory was of the nature of an emergency effort to lift themselves into group membership with contemporaries. The revolutionary and destructive attitude seemed to base itself upon a conviction of impending calamity and necessary unsuccess in a hostile world. *Emergency, crisis, drive—*but they were very unhappy people. At the time of which I write, such persons were usually communists.

More recently, when doing some work in collaboration with a medical clinician of Boston, I happened upon a case essentially similar, though driven by circumstance in another direction. The patient was a man of powerful build who had successfully held many "strong arm" jobs. I call him the "gunman," not because he had ever fallen to the level of gangster work, but because he had lived in very rough society and had a habit when I first knew him of carrying a "gat" in his left armpit. Amongst other ills which had brought him to the physician was an attitude of extreme puzzlement that he could not obtain employment. He claimed that his first prospects of a job were always bright, that he was always one of the first applicants to be interviewed, but that somehow the interview always "went wrong." He did not at first attribute this failure to anything in himself; he was inclined to play with the idea of some conspiracy against him. He clearly had no conception of the threatening attitude he adopted—even at the beginning of his hospital interview—an attitude in itself sufficient, I am sure, to discourage any prospective employer.

This case was remarkable in its outcome—even more dramatic than the other—since it was one of those comparatively rare situations which clear up suddenly by means of what the literary call a "blinding flash" of insight. That this phenomenon is not unknown to psychologists is evidenced by Piaget's discussion of the *croyance déclenchée* in children[3] or by Freud's discussion of "abreaction," which is in some respects similar.[4] This case, then, was unlike the ordinary because in the first interview the patient came to realize that the greater part of his trouble was due to his aggressive, indeed truculent, attitude to a world that he believed to be uniformly hostile to him. There had to be other interviews to help him work out the aggressive pattern in detail in order

[3]Jean Piaget, *The Child's Conception of the World* (New York: Harcourt, Brace and Company, 1929), introduction.

[4]Sigmund Freud, *Selected Papers on Hysteria and Other Psychoneuroses* (New York and Washington: Nervous and Mental Disease Publishing Company, 1920), pp. 1-13.

that he might control it, but the effective conviction was released almost at once. After recovery he wrote his physician an unusual letter of thanks, from which I am permitted to quote some paragraphs. At the head of his letter he places a title, "The Fighting Cock and a Hostile World. New Life." He begins:

Fifteen years of plain unadulterated Hell with a capital H. A Hell of my own making, the price one pays for being a fighter, a fighter who has gone beyond the rules of the game and has carried it to almost a fanatical degree. The misery, loneliness, and the helpless feeling one gets trying to fight alone a hostile world, cannot be put into words.

His history he sketches briefly:

No one in whom I could confide, no one that I might call a true friend. The things I loved most, and those that I loved, were taken away. There was not one thing that I could really call my own. Defence after defence I threw up to ward off more hurt, retreating ever retreating into my shell. Till finally I became a snarling animal at bay. The few people I did know slowly left me, people shunned me on the street. . . I became suspicious of everyone. I looked for trouble to present itself most anywhere, and looking for it I found plenty. I tried to smash my way through life's barriers, crushing those that opposed me, fighting, snarling, to retain my place in the world. In doing so I created a world of hate, which finally overpowered me.

Towards the end of a four-page letter of graphic description, he says:

I wish I might express in words just what I have been through, the pain, the loneliness, the heartbreaks and torture of fighting alone. Then and only then could one understand to a small degree the gratitude . . . To change from a snarling animal at bay to once again a man that is at least safe to have around is . . . little short of a miracle.

When describing these or similar cases on other occasions I have sometimes heard such phrases as "paranoid personality" applied in comment. And indeed this phrase is admirably descriptive; the difficulty is that *it carries an implication of organic dysfunction or pathology* as the root of the trouble. Now unquestionably there are cases that are organically determined; but all paranoid attitudes do not necessarily originate in somatic pathology. If it were so, all primitive peoples, all children, and indeed every one of us would be pathological. For there is no one who has not experienced something of the attitude of the artisan or the gunman as a passing phenomenon under sufficient provocation—*and especially when young.* In addition to this, I have described seven cases, two in some detail: of the seven, two chanced to consult medical colleagues about some other and minor ill and were given attention for their major disability; both patients made an excellent recovery. It is surely most probable, from the evidence, that these were both instances of failure to achieve sanity. Some grave defects in their early surrounding left them almost completely unconditioned for a life of social participation. And their rebellion against a hostile world is no more than a necessary symptom of their social ignorance and incapacity.

Indeed it may be said of all seven, that in listening

to their self-history one gradually but inevitably derived the impression that they could not be other than they were. It was not difficult to sort out the actual fact from the rationalized explanations in what they said and so to arrive at this conclusion. Beyond this, they were like the rest of us. They saw the world as we do, without hallucination, even if they described it differently. Their capacity for continuous thinking was above the average; their thinking indeed was too continuous. Their capacity for logical thinking was unusual; they liked nothing better than tortuous, endless, quasi-logical argument.

At this point I realize that my illustrations, chosen for their relative simplicity, may be somewhat misleading. Every case in greater or less degree displays the hate-hostility-destruction attitude. And this fact might seem to identify obsession in general with one special manifestation of it. That this interpretation is far from my intention, the sequel will show. It is a fact of observation that every obsessive regards the social world about him as remote, strange, hostile, and that we ourselves in any passing mood of obsession echo the same assumption. But the individual response to this mood is far more often characterized by fear and excessive precaution than by an opposing and aggressive hostility. The more closely one studies the recorded cases of Janet and Freud, the more evident does it seem that there are two varieties of obsessives: *frightened people*[5] and *destroyers*, the for-

---

[5]See also "Frightened People" in the appendix.

mer more commonly encountered than the latter. Dr. J. S. Plant, in his recent New Jersey studies, has suggested a similar classification. He distinguishes between "panic" and "rebellion" in the typical responses—an almost identical distinction made in a somewhat different human situation.[6] The one attitude implies "the world is dangerous, I must be careful"; the other, "the world is hostile, let me attack it."

Further discussion of this distinction is better postponed, for there is an inference that must be stated before ending this chapter. This is that, from the point of view of clinical psychology, everything a person says or does must be regarded as an item in a context—the context being the personal history and present social situation of the individual. This will seem to be in direct contradiction of almost all that is taught by the expositors of those university subjects of study that circle vaguely around the humanities. And indeed it is so—for the university method of taking every assertion *au pied de la lettre* and examining it for its logical reference and adequacy, though perhaps excellent for intellectual training, is exceedingly bad for intelligent practice. I do not mean that such instruction should be banished from the classroom; the student who follows it faithfully *gains something in control of thinking, something in capacity for accurate statement. But he who seeks to understand and live contentedly with his fellows must*

---

[6]James S. Plant, *Personality and the Cultural Pattern* (New York: The Commonwealth Fund, 1937), pp. 99-105.

begin from where their thinking actually is and not from where the textbooks say it should be. In the case quoted of the "atheist" the usual method of conversational approach to the individual was through the mental fog of pseudological religious argument. This approach achieved nothing but exasperation for both participants in the discussion, whereas the slightest attention to context—the history and immediate situation of the individual—instantly showed the alleged atheism to be no more than a symptom of an actual and present disability. So also with the six "destroyers": they were heavily intrenched against the usual approach that sought to controvert the Marxian logic—indeed they were completely proof against any such attack. But in every instance, study of the personal context showed the intellectualist discussion to be secondary to, and no more than symptomatic of, a destroyer attitude that expressed a badly damaged relationship with other persons. This does not imply that every person who professes interest in such doctrines is mentally ill; on the contrary, the diagnosis has no validity beyond the cases actually cited. It does imply that a clinical psychology must ignore completely the truth or falsity (or other value) of what is said in interview and must look for the significance of all statements in the situation of the person that makes them. Consequently the simple rules for the conduct of any clinical interview, whether medical or sociological, are as follows:

1. Give your whole attention to the person interviewed, and make it evident that you are doing so.

2. Listen—don't talk.

3. Never argue, never give advice.

4. Listen to:
   (a) What he wants to say.
   (b) What he does not want to say.
   (c) What he cannot say without help.

5. As you listen, plot out tentatively and for subsequent correction the pattern that is being set before you. To test this, occasionally summarize what has been said and present it for comment. Always do this with caution—that is, abbreviate and clarify but do not add or "twist."

6. Remember that everything said must be considered a personal confidence and not divulged to anyone. (This does not prevent discussion of a situation between professional colleagues. Nor does it prevent some form of public report when due precaution has been taken.)

The need for such simple rules will become obvious after we have given some time to sufficiently detailed study of the clinical findings of Janet.

C

II

HYSTERIA AND HYPNOSIS

When the development of clinical psychology is fully documented by historians, it will be found that the modern impulse to interest did not take its rise mainly in psychiatry. The critical interest of the psychiatrist was obviously required, but it was in the ordinary practice of medicine that the problem had its origin. Janet traces the development to the controversy between *fluidists* and *animists*, which was a variant of the enduring medical disagreement as to the organic or mental origin of hysteria.[1] Milne Bramwell traces it to a rise of interest in hypnotism after the Abbé Faria had returned from a visit to the East.[2] English medicine was roused to critical consideration of the possible value of hypnosis as part of the technical equipment of the physician by general practitioners such as Esdaile and Elliotson,

[1] Pierre Janet, *Les Médications Psychologiques* (Paris: Librairie Felix Alcan, 1918), vol. I; translated from the French by Eden and Cedar Paul, *Psychological Healing* (New York: Macmillan Company, 1925), I, 159.

[2] J. Milne Bramwell, *Hypnotism, Its History, Practice and Theory* (London: William Rider & Son, Ltd., 1921), pp. 3 ff.

and later by Milne Bramwell and Lloyd Tuckey. Throughout Europe in the mid-nineteenth century there was a sudden fury of interest in this question; eminent physicians who supported the use of hypnosis were to be found in France, Switzerland, Germany, Holland, and elsewhere. The medical journals contained numerous papers on hysteria; many textbooks were published and are still obtainable. Thus the study of mental hygiene began as an inquiry into hypnosis and hysteria.

But all this activity and interest led nowhere until Dr. James Braid was roused to investigation. Before Braid, the medical interest had directed itself mainly to questions of the possible utility of hypnosis in minor surgery or in the control of hysterical attacks. It was Braid who first asked what the curious hypnotic condition is and began to take interest in it on its own account. At first he took the view that it was an abnormal condition of the central nervous system induced by fixed gazing, definitely an organic variant and somewhat akin to sleep. It was he who coined the words *hypnosis, hypnotism*, and so on, at this stage. Later he developed an alternate theory that hypnosis was not organic but mental—a condition induced by concentration of attention upon a monotonous or unchanging object. In support of this view, which he believed himself to have established experimentally, he coined the word *monoideism*. But his first word held the field and has passed into ordinary use.

Braid's work attracted the attention of Charcot, the eminent neurologist of the Salpêtrière Hospital in Paris; and with this stimulus the modern development of psychopathology began. Charcot in 1882 demonstrated the possibility of producing by hypnotic suggestion, in those who were able to achieve the somnambulic state, the exact symptoms of hysteria. That is, he was able to suggest to a somnambule that on waking he would not be able to use, for example, one or other arm. When aroused, the patient would exhibit all the usual symptoms of hysterical anesthesia and hysterical paralysis, so-called, in the limb in question. This led to the suspicion that hypnotizability was a symptom of one form of hysteria. And it was at this point that Pierre Janet took up the research.

It is the fashion in these days to dismiss, somewhat cavalierly, the work of Janet as something that has been superseded by Freudian and other developments. This is partly due, no doubt, to the fact that his major publications on psychopathology have never been translated into English, so that even the medical world is for the most part ignorant of his patient and accurate observations over a period of fifty years. It is also due to a peculiar characteristic of many Freudian psychologists: the fact that they refuse to read anything whatever outside the pale of psychoanalysis. It is as if they feared that their faith might be shattered. The outcome is unfortunate, for there is no real conflict between the observations of Janet and Freud. Indeed they work in different parts of the same field so that their researches are mutually complementary; and any person trained in the findings of one only is probably committed to incomplete understanding. I hope to make this clear as the discussion is developed.

Janet's original work, first published fifty years ago, was based upon careful and detailed studies of a number of hysterical patients.[3] His remarkable findings attracted the attention of William James. Those who are unable to read Janet in the original will find a brief but useful summary in *The Principles of Psychology*.[4] The first question to be faced was that of the significance of the anesthetic (or hyperesthetic) localities in the skin sensations of the hysteric. These insensitive spots had been recognized in the Middle Ages. They were then described as "devil's seals" and were supposed to indicate the witch. Any place where the devil had laid his unholy hand during a midnight witches' Sabbath became anesthetic; so ran the fable, supported in the popular estimate by the fact that those other powers of mediumship and trance possessed by some so-called witches were equally symptoms of hysteria. Thus "devils' seals" and other supposed stigmata of witchcraft may have occurred frequently in the same person. Until Janet, it had always been assumed by medical inquiry that this type of anesthesia must be

---

[3]Pierre Janet, *L'Automatisme Psychologique* (Paris: Librairie Felix Alcan, 1889).

[4]William James (London: Macmillan and Co. Limited, 1890), especially chapter VIII of vol. I, and chapter XXVII of vol. II.

more or less of a kind with that which indicates
definite organic injury.

"Hysteria," Charcot used to say, "is a mental malady"; but
this phrase which he so liked to repeat remained for him and
his contemporaries a mere formula. In reality they continued to assume that this disability is a complex of
symptoms analogous to those which characterize injuries
of the nerve-centres. They studied hysteria exactly as they
studied these other ills and without adequate precaution.
And they did not bother to examine closely the ideas and
sentiments of the patient.[5]

This oversimplified hypothesis involved neurologists and physicians in considerable difficulty, for
in an hysterical patient the right side of the body may
be apparently paralyzed on one day but the left side
on the day after. Furthermore, the usual neurological
tests did not indicate any injury or lesion of the
appropriate nerves or nerve centers. Such observations inevitably led to suspicion of imposture, malin-
gering, or "skrimshanking." These facts tended to
induce in physicians generally an attitude of im-
patience with hysterical patients, which occasionally
showed itself in great harshness of treatment.

The quotation cited above from Janet will show
that his first concern was to develop adequate observation and description. His rejection of the oversimplified neurological hypothesis does not mean that
he excluded all possibility of the relation of hysterical
symptoms to an actual organic dysfunction. On the

---

[5]Pierre Janet, *Les Névroses* (Paris: Ernest Flammarion, 1909),
p. 325.

contrary, his attitude is to be described as cautious, as a claim that accurate observation of the hysteric should be much extended before coming to any conclusion at all. For he discovered that, while the capacity for having sensation and responding to it is locally undiminished in the apparently paralyzed arm of an hysterical patient, nevertheless the awareness of sensation and the direction of response are not included in that part of the patient's mentality that is communicating with his physician. His first observations were to the effect that the general awareness (that is to say, of surrounding) of the hysterics with whom he talked was in a sense much narrower than in the normal person. The patient Lucie, for example, would talk freely to him but ignored completely the presence of others in the room. She not only disregarded the ordinary interruptions of persons coming and going, she was also quite immune to any interruption. Standing by her one might ask questions, only to find that she would continue the main conversation and not notice the questions. One might even shout in her ear without any response, without deflecting for a moment her primary preoccupation. This patient had an anesthetic hand and arm—hysterical paralysis.

Janet began with very simple experiments. For example, he put her pince-nez glasses in her apparently unusable hand. The hand at once pinched them open and raised them towards her face. When they came into her field of vision, she said in apparent

astonishment, "Why, I have eyeglasses in my hand."
In several of these patients Janet developed the capacity for separate response, until it was possible to conduct two conversations with them simultaneously.
The patient's main attention was held in conversation by someone, while Janet whispered questions to her from behind the chair in which she was seated. By practice the anesthetic hand was enabled to write intelligible answers to the whispered questions without any interruption of the main conversation. Indeed the primary, or normal, self remained apparently totally unaware of both the whispered question and the written answer. This is the so-called double personality, or alternating personality, of the true hysteric—a striking and characteristic phenomenon. Janet termed this method the method of *distraction*, and he began to speak of this characteristic splitting of a complex personality into primary and secondary selves as *dissociation*.

This word, dissociation, is intended descriptively and is used by him to denote two observations: first, in hysteria there seems to be a considerable disjunction between parts of the sensory field, so that there is a diminution of their mutual awareness; and, second, this disjunction seems to find reflection in an equivalent lack of relation between the various systems of acquired response, these latter usually deemed in their normal synthesis to constitute what is known as personality.[6]

---

[6]For further discussion of this topic, see Chapter III.

Janet was able to demonstrate very neatly the clear-cut division between these fragmented systems of response. On one occasion he told the patient Lucie while in hypnosis that he was about to place cards with numbers on them in her lap and that she would not see on waking those numbers that were multiples of three. Having waked her, he placed six cards in her lap, the numbers two, four, twelve, eighteen, nine, ten. He asked, "How many cards?" "Three," replied Lucie I, the primary self. "What numbers on them?" "Four, two, ten." The instructions had been obeyed and the threes were not seen. Getting some other person to engage Lucie's primary attention, he whispered to Lucie II, the secondary self, "How many cards has Lucie in her lap?" "Three," wrote the anesthetic arm and hand. "What numbers?" "Twelve, eighteen, nine." The secondary, or dissociated, self had seen only those cards ignored by the primary self. An interesting incident occurred at this point. At the moment when Lucie II looked at the cards, Lucie I paused in her conversation, put her hand to her head, and ejaculated, "Oh! I cannot see!" This experiment demonstrated very clearly the so-called dissociation, the *weakened integrity* of awareness and response. It also demonstrated the complementary nature of the dissociate fragments.

These observations Janet repeated in a number of cases at the Salpêtrière and in private practice; he was thus enabled to extend usefully the description of two facts generally known to, but little understood by, medicine, namely, *hypnosis* and *suggestion*. The word suggestion is used ordinarily to cover so wide a range of human situations that its specific meaning dwindles almost to zero. A scholar may suggest the works of a certain authority to a student for consultation; any one of us who has been reassured by his personal physician is apt to describe his feeling of relief as the effect of suggestion. The term has unfortunately been used almost as vaguely in medicine and frequently conveys a totally erroneous implication, that situations described by the same word must be identical in some essential particular. This is not what Janet means by "suggestion": *he uses the word to describe a specific character of hysteria which has not been observed in the normal organism or in other mental disability.*

Those persons who suffer the diminished integrity of awareness and response that Janet describes as hysteria exhibit also another characteristic symptom. The inferior dissociated fragment, the so-called secondary self, displays a curious immediate relationship with actual organic function, which would seem to imply a definite diminution of normal cortical mediation or inhibition. This I can illustrate from an industrial experience. Some years ago while engaged upon a factory inquiry, my colleagues and I had tentatively developed the opinion that a certain worker, a man of about twenty-seven, was a Janet hysteric and probably did much of his work in the hypnotic condition. One day while at work he slightly scratched his hand and fell into a condition of primitive panic entirely disproportionate to the negligible injury. This occurrence seemed to confirm the opinion that he had been doing his work while in a somnambulic condition. In the small factory clinic where he was raging he was accordingly asked to sit down and relax. He did so and passed instantly into deep hypnosis; while he sat passively thus, he was extensively reassured. When awakened he had completely lost his panic and was no longer concerned about his injury; the reassurance had been addressed not to the primary, but to the appropriate secondary, self. He returned to work and showed no further signs of alarm.

Dr. S. D. Ludlum,[7] who was collaborating in the industrial inquiry, volunteered a thorough medical examination of this worker and, since the patient asked it, of his wife also. The examination confirmed the diagnosis of hysteria; it was also discovered in conversation that the patient suffered an extravagant fear that his wife, to whom he was devotedly attached, had contracted a malignant disease. Medical examination of the wife showed that this fear was fortunately without justification; and it was therefore arranged, as an experiment, that the appropriate reassurance should be given to the patient while he was in the somnambulic condition. He was given a

---

[7]Professor of neuropsychiatry, Graduate School of Medicine, University of Pennsylvania.

barium meal, and two observers watched his stomach in the fluorescent screen while the communication was made. At first his stomach was large and completely quiescent. Two sentences were spoken to him. The first was, "You have been afraid that your wife might have cancer." When this was said his external appearance did not change in any particular, but his stomach went into active movement. The next sentence was, "You need have no fear, your wife has no serious disease." Again, there was no external evidence that he had heard, but his stomach instantly ceased movement and became again quiescent. It is this extraordinarily direct relationship between the secondary self of an hysteric, the self that appears in hypnosis, and the organic functions proper that Janet indicates when he speaks of suggestion. It is this relationship which manifests itself in the shifting anesthesias and false paralyses of hysteria. Let any circumstance suggest a disability to the secondary, or dissociate, awareness and at once the disability appears as a fact accomplished. No discussion with, or reassurance to, the primary awareness will affect it in the least. This is the outstanding difference between suggestibility in an hysteric and what we sometimes call suggestibility in ourselves.

A similar comment may be made with respect to the hypnotic state. We have observed in several industrial instances that an hysteric of the Janet type frequently does his daily routine work in the hypnotic condition without ever realizing the fact. It is only persons who frequently make use of hypnosis in this fashion (in other words, without realizing it) who can be hypnotized.[8] In making this statement I am using the word *hypnosis* as Janet and Charcot used it to denote true somnambulism. It is only the deepest condition of somnambulism which presents the typical characters of hypnosis—posthypnotic suggestion, organic involvement, and the like. The hypnotic condition consequently cannot be imposed upon any person who does not ordinarily make use of it; that is, it can only be achieved by the true hysteric. The old-fashioned superstition that "power of will," or a "magnetic eye," in the so-called hypnotist may be responsible is nonsense.

A girl worker in an eastern factory complained to her foreman that she had no objection to the factory physician talking to her as she worked at her machine, but she thought he had no right to make an incision in her side while she was at work—and in the presence of others. This complaint was heard by her fellow workers and induced in them and in the foreman considerable alarm. She was brought into hospital—with the suggestion that "she has dementia praecox." It was discovered almost at once that she was hypnotizable, and there followed an interesting period in which the two selves had to be talked to alternately. She had been accustomed to drop into somnambulism while working and had failed to distinguish between the dream states, which seemed to

---

[8]Pierre Janet, *Les Névroses*, pp. 273-274.

be vividly present to her, and the actuality about her. With some coaching she effected the distinction and came to realize that the incidents she had described had not really happened. This type of hypnotic state is clearly confined to the dissociate hysteric. Indeed, Janet's researches give one a descriptive answer to the question of why hypnosis is hypnosis. *The diminution of the primary awareness as an hysteric relaxes or takes up repetitive work does not promote a balanced relaxation as in the normal person.* On the contrary, it yields control to the dissociate set of responses, the so-called secondary self, so making possible the active conversations and other phenomena that occur in hypnosis without disturbing the slumber of the primary self.

In other instances, the dissociate fragments will sometimes participate in the same conversation and ignore each other completely—which those who hear it are unable to do. A Methodist lay preacher was brought to a physician for consultation by the elders of his church. He was renowned for his eloquence in sermons, but had taken to inserting a high, thin, derisive "ee-ee-ee-ee" after his most eloquent periods. The elders had remonstrated without effect, except that whispered blasphemies began to be substituted for the mere "ee-ee-ee." These whispers unfortunately could be heard by those nearest to him in the church—hence, the consultation. On one occasion, when I was present, he was being questioned about the general circumstances of his youth and upbringing. Two physicians were present and the discussion turned upon the events of adolescence and puberty. He was asked if he remembered any sex preoccupations during the adolescent period. He answered, "No sir; I never thought about those things." This was immediately followed by a derisive whisper, "Bloody liar." This considerably discomposed his professional audience but had no visible effect upon the patient. It was as if he had not heard it.

There is still another form of hysteria which again illustrates this curious ignorance in the primary self of what its secondary dissociate is doing. These cases are the so-called fugues, in the course of which the patient leaves his accustomed haunts and lives a completely different life elsewhere. Neither he nor his new associates seem to suspect anything unusual or abnormal in him. Janet describes several instances of this kind;[9] William James cites the case of the Rev. Ansel Bourne. The case I quote was a transient hysteria, which belongs logically to a group that is discussed on the pages immediately following[10] but which I insert here because the subject's disability took the form of a fugue.

The patient was in a mental hospital listed as a case of mild melancholia. A medical colleague and I were asked to see him because he was said to be recovering after some months under medical care. In the early period of the war of 1914 the patient had

[9]*Les Névroses*, pp. 242 ff.
[10]See pp. 39 ff.

disappeared completely when on his way by train to enlist. About twelve months later he appeared at his home shabbily dressed and completely unable to give an account of what he had been doing. He had awakened one morning, several hundred miles from the city in which he lived, and found to his astonishment that he had been working for months on a farm as a laborer. His mental mood was definitely melancholic but for a time he lived with his family—wife, son, and daughter—who were earning comfortable incomes. Then one day he arranged to meet his wife in the city, missed her, and walked steadily northwards for a week, coming to himself in another city one hundred miles away. During this time he had effectively performed all the small routines of living, paying for his room and meals, answering questions, and so on, without arousing any suspicion of abnormality. On another occasion, and again when meeting his wife, he walked two hundred miles southwards and on coming to himself was again utterly unable to remember the events of the preceding days. It was after this that he voluntarily put himself under medical care.

At the time when we saw him the hysterical dissociation, or fragmentation of his awareness of surrounding, had for the most part disappeared. I do not remember that we even tried to induce hypnosis. I think not, for the reason that he was able to tell us in interview the preoccupations of both his primary and secondary dissociates sufficiently well. His story, briefly, was that of personal failure. He had been a skilled mechanic, a foreman of a department in a prosperous firm. An admirable husband and father, he had always provided well for his family; he owned the small house in which they lived, had given the best education obtainable to his son and daughter, and had considerable savings. Then the firm for which he had always worked went out of business, and he was unable to get another job. He felt the change of status very keenly and made heroic efforts to get work—even the work of a laborer—but was unsuccessful. After some time his wife, a vigorous and capable person, took a job in a department store to help the family fortunes. It happened that she developed an unexpected flair for the kind of work she was given and was rapidly promoted until she became a buyer for the store. As a buyer, she earned far more than her husband had ever made even in his most prosperous years, and thus became the family support. The patient meanwhile found no work and was accustomed to sit at home brooding over the change. It was after a few years spent thus that he developed the hysterical fugue. Extensive "talking over" the situation helped him to complete his recovery and he left the hospital.

The war of 1914 developed a great number of cases of transient hysteria, described usually as "shell shock." I call these cases transient, because just as the conditions of trench warfare provoked in some unknown fashion these hysterias, so also relief from war conditions was in many instances sufficient to promote recovery. Some recovered rapidly without professional aid other than a hospital bed and sufficient sleep; in other instances the persistence of specific fears delayed recovery until psychopathological aid was required; still others did not recover at all—these were frequently the older men. It is of the second group of cases that I speak here, those who were in need of skilled aid to complete recovery. The usual method adopted was that of hypnosis. In hypnosis it was possible in the majority of cases to reassure the dissociate fragment directly—to persuade it that the war was over, that the organic disability was unnecessary; for the secondary self is not persuaded even by those changes of external circumstance to which the primary self has apparently adapted. This inaccessibility of the secondary self to ordinary communication has been already mentioned in the discussion of suggestibility.

It is this inaccessibility of the conscious fragment in control of organic symptoms that Janet discusses under the title of the "fixed ideas" of hysteria; Freud refers to it in his "Preliminary Communication" as existing "like a foreign body" in the total conscious attitude of the patient, which continues long after its incidence to "influence like a new causative factor."[11] This finds illustration in the case of a highly regarded sergeant of cavalry in Palestine who after

---

[11]Sigmund Freud, *Selected Papers on Hysteria and Other Psychoneuroses,* pp. 4-8.

several years of meritorious service suddenly went amok, released the horses, attacked his comrades, and had to be put under constraint. He went to sleep and on awaking remembered nothing of the incident. He was invalided to base hospital, then sent home. During the subsequent months when he was under observation the dissociation developed. On afternoons when he had leave he was apt to board a public conveyance and later find himself at the terminus without any recollection of the journey. His physicians had attempted to discover directly the possible emotional sources of the original incident in camp. These inquiries had proved fruitless, a complete amnesia guarded the primary consciousness from any recollection of the event. Under hypnosis, which he achieved instantly and easily, it was suggested to him that he should go back to the original situation in Palestine and express what he was thinking. He began at once to perspire, to curse the dust, the heat, the flies, and to tear at his collar. As Janet remarks of his cases, it was an extraordinarily realistic exhibition; watching in the cool hospital ward, one almost began to feel the heat and discomfort oneself. Immediately after he was wakened, his physician began to rehearse to him what he had said in hypnosis. In many war cases the dissociation was so recent and the patient so healthy in other respects that a direct attack upon the dysfunction was sometimes effective. Some of the most interesting results, indeed, were thus effected without the aid of hypnosis. This I shall presently illustrate.

Another case was that of a young man in the early twenties who had been shot through the upper arm. The ulnar nerve had been severed and there had been a surgical resection. At the time when he was referred by his surgeon to a physician, his symptoms were inability to move the flexed third and small fingers of his left hand ("wrist-drop") and excessive tenderness (hyperesthesia) in the locality of the wound. He also complained of mental confusion such that he was unable to do the clerical work to which he had returned after being invalided. He was actually losing weight. The first symptom—the flexed fingers—was appropriate; not until the ulnar nerve had restored itself could control return. The wrist-drop was organically unnecessary, so also the hyperesthesia. This last so distressed him that he wore a padded metal shield to guard his arm from chance contacts. His physician found that he was hypnotizable and began accordingly to make the appropriate suggestions when he was in the somnambulic condition. In three days the patient presented the metal shield to his doctor and proudly fingered his arm to show that the extra sensitivity had vanished. In a week he was able to hold his hand up from the wrist for a moment or two. In three weeks he had lost all symptoms other than the flexed fingers; his mental confusion had disappeared and he had gained over fourteen pounds in weight. In this case as in others it cannot be claimed that the psychopathological work of the physician was wholly responsible for the recovery of the patient. It is doubtful whether psychopathology alone has ever *cured* hysteria. When an hysteric recovers with dramatic suddenness, it is more likely that the organic interference responsible for the dissociate integrity of awareness has diminished or disappeared. Nevertheless, as in certain cases of hemiplegia, re-education is required to restore the function.

The most dramatic instance of recovered function that I have seen occurred in a military hospital for "shell-shock" soldiers. A patient was sent in one afternoon from another hospital. His history was that for two years he had been losing capacity to use his left forearm and hand; finally it had become useless to him. He also suffered "fits" or "spells." His medical officers, after many careful examinations, had come to believe that he was affected with an obscure hysteria. He was intelligent and cooperative; he had not previously been examined for hysteria. The interview that followed—without any attempt to induce hypnosis—was interesting. Over two years before when he was going through his military training, the large camp in which he was living had suffered an epidemic of cerebrospinal meningitis. The patient contracted the disease and was very ill for eight weeks. Then he recovered, and without any loss of muscular function. He was given leave, which he spent at home, returning later to camp to resume his training. He returned to a camp which had become afflicted with a species of panic by reason of the epidemic. Before his return, the patient had not known what the name of his disease meant; now he learned three things from his comrades, all of which he dutifully accepted. The three supposed facts were these: first, that he had had meningitis; second, that those who have had meningitis sooner or later lose the use of a limb; third, that they finally "go mad." These supposed facts were a heavy load for an unlettered private soldier to carry. His first attack occurred, he said, after an afternoon spent in practicing trench digging; it occurred that evening in cantonments. After recovery from a "spell," he noticed that the fingers of his left hand seemed stiff. Questioned more closely, he said that the field in which the digging took place had been christened "Meningitis Flats" by his comrades. Asked why, he said they believed that those who turned up the earth there were likely to contract the epidemic disease. His second attack occurred on a military transport bound for France. What time of day? Afternoon. What had he been doing? Having a bath. Before that? Listening to the fellows talk. What were they talking about? The aftereffects of meningitis. And so on through the history of the earlier attacks, each one tracing to a strong suggestion of the certainty of disability as a consequence of his illness. He had never discussed the matter with his physicians, who had continued to give him a clean bill of health in other respects. When it became clear to him that there had never been any evidence of neurological damage, he was asked whether he was suffering from the actual aftereffects or from fear of such aftereffects. He thought a moment and then replied, "From fear, sir." Asked if there was any reason why he should not use his left hand and arm, he said slowly, "No, sir." The medical officer in charge put a pin on the bed coverlet and said, "Pick it up." He picked it up with the unusable left hand. The interview occupied twenty-three minutes. As we left the room, he was lifting various objects on the small table beside him and replacing them.

It is interesting that, whereas the military cases tended to make good recoveries, there are no available records to show that many of the classical civilian cases did so. Janet holds his case records but they have not been published as records; on one occasion he told me that a number of his most interesting hysterias had ultimately died of phthisis. If it is true that the younger patients tend to recover with medical and psychopathological aid, this would seem to put them in the same category as the military cases. To this topic I shall return briefly in another chapter; in the meantime, and by way of summary, it will be well to restate Janet's conclusions.

In his own summary in *Les Névroses*,[12] Janet points to the *retraction* (*rétrécissement*) of the field of conscious awareness of surrounding and to *dissociation* as the distinguishing characters of hysteria.

---

[12]Pages 317-345.

He admits at once[13] that a dissociation of functions might be claimed equally as a character of dementia; but in dementia one finds a mere "dust heap" of ideas, habits, instincts replacing the systematic constructions of the normal. The dissociation of hysteria, he says, is distinguished from mental deterioration of a dementia type by the fact that "in spite of the dissociation the function itself remains almost undamaged." Hysteria must accordingly be regarded from this point of view as "a malady of the personality." The dissociate functions are undamaged; but the capacity to hold together multiple functions, both natural and derived, in a single complex act of perception is gravely diminished during the course of an hysteria. Furthermore, the systems of ideas and functions thus emancipated tend to take on an almost independent existence and development, and it is to this fact of observation that most of the extraordinary symptoms of hysteria—hypnosis, suggestibility, alternating personality—must be traced. These clinical findings lead Janet to state explicitly the implications of his researches for a psychology of the normal mind. These implications I shall consider in the next chapter.

---

[13]Page 343.

III

THE COMPLEXITY
OF THE ATTENTIVE ACT

Hysteria is, as Janet says, so "extraordinary a malady" of the human organism that no useful purpose outside of medicine would be served by studying it were it not that his observations led him to reëxamine, and closely, the processes of perception in the normal person. In doing this, he is led to state an hypothesis which possesses great importance for all psychological study. Our conscious awareness of surrounding, he points out, is an exceedingly complex fact, which can be described only as a balanced relation among an indefinite number of perceptions. Our mental life, he says, "consists not only of a succession of phenomena coming one after the other and forming a long series . . . but each of these successive states is in reality a complex state; it contains a multitude of elementary facts and owes its apparent unity to synthesis alone, to the equilibrium of all these elements." In at least three of his best known books he insists upon this description as *essential to all accurate psychological observation.*[1]

Almost all the major academic psychologists are to some extent aware of this; some even state it quite explicitly. Titchener, for example, in his *Outline of Psychology* begins by describing our mental awareness of surrounding as "a sum of simultaneous processes . . . which run their course in time together."[2] Bosanquet in discussing "the general nature of psychical events" says, "the presentations which occupy the focus of attention at any moment are really the smallest part of what the mind has present to it; there is a field which is occupied by presentations which are not in focus, and therefore not discriminated, and the whole state of consciousness takes its colouring very much from these."[3] He goes on to point out that in every person's awareness there are certain "permanent and many habitual elements" which go far to "bind consciousness as one whole." It is to be observed that these statements go far beyond a mere assertion of the complexity of our awareness of surrounding at any given moment. In addition to this, Bosanquet makes two claims: first, that capacity to respond at a given moment depends upon the system-

---

[1]Pierre Janet, *L'Automatisme Psychologique* (9th ed.; Paris: Librairie Felix Alcan, 1921), p. 194; *L'État Mental des Hystériques* (Paris: Felix Alcan, 1911), p. 425; *Les Névroses* (Paris: Ernest Flammarion, 1909), pp. 338-339.

[2]E. B. Titchener (New York: Macmillan Company, 1898), p. 11.

[3]B. Bosanquet, *Psychology of the Moral Self* (London: Macmillan and Co., Limited, 1904), p. 18.

atic interrelation of the various elements in the complexity; and, second, that the relative involvement in any specific response is relatively small—and there are certain "permanent and many habitual elements" which continue almost unchanged through a series of such responses. Titchener supports this by reiteration of the phrase that "meaning, psychologically, is always context";[4] in other words, the nature of a specific response is determined not merely by some item in the external or sensory situation but by the whole developed system of capacity for response.

Now Bosanquet, once he has called attention to this complexity, proceeds to ignore it altogether; there are many psychologists who follow this lead. For half a century the academic psychology has occupied itself for the most part with studies of attentive thinking, that is, experiments with special acts of attention. The assumption is that the whole complex biochemical, neurological, personal balance will maintain itself in such fashion that the only difference from moment to moment is that required by some particular response to a particular stimulus in the surrounding. This assumption is both justifiable and useful, provided it is not forgotten that capacity to attend depends upon a multiplicity of other determinants. But for Janet as clinician this assumption is not possible. The clinician is asked to investigate personal situations characterized by the diminution

---

[4]E. B. Titchener, *A Text-Book of Psychology* (New York: Macmillan Company, 1921), p. 367.

or distortion of normal awareness and normal response. In such instances the many determinants other than the response (or act of attention) itself become important and must be carefully and systematically examined. The services of medicine, neurology, and psychiatry may all be required in cases of special difficulty. And indeed the special skills that these words represent have all been brought to bear upon the medical histories that Janet reports.

It is only after he has been assured by medicine and neurology that there is no observable gross organic unbalance in his patients that Janet is free to investigate in new directions. And he proceeds to make observations of two kinds that have not been sufficiently developed by medicine or psychology. These two may be named as follows: first, the capacity of an organism to maintain its full complexity of balanced relationship within itself and with the world about it; and, second, the capacity of an organism to *complicate* its responses. The latter has been studied by psychology but usually as if unrelated to the former.

Everyone in these days is familiar with the use of a diagram of the "reflex arc" to give students a first simple idea of the structure and function of a nervous system. A sense organ or sensory surface is depicted as the source of stimulus from which an afferent nerve leads to a nerve cell or center; this center is connected by nerves with another such center from which proceeds an efferent nerve to muscle or other response—a synapse or so may be thrown in for good measure. The diagram does give some idea of the structural unit of a nervous system but is the source of many misleading conceptions of nervous function. A student who assumes an independent reflex automatism in the action of such an arc tends also to assume that a collection of such arcs constitutes a nervous system. Any student who thinks thus is likely to underestimate the mutual dependence of the constituent parts of an organic equilibrium and to underestimate also the balanced relation of nervous with other organic functions and with the external sensory world. Now very simple organisms do not possess a nervous system; and when a nervous system does appear in even a relatively simple organism, the biologist knows that he is already inspecting a natural contrivance for the maintenance of integrity of response. Sherrington's experimental work shows that the organism as a whole exercises what might be termed a permissive function upon the responses of even the lower level reflex arcs.[5] Technically this is described as the facilitation of one set of activities and the inhibition of others; the system is responding to stimulus as a whole and is no mere additive group of reflex elements. This balanced relationship strongly affects even the sensations from receptors. Head, in his studies of injuries to the cerebral cortex during the war of 1914-1918, showed that in certain instances

---

[5]C. S. Sherrington, *The Integrative Action of the Nervous System* (New York: Charles Scribner's Sons, 1906), pp. 387-393.

the effect of destruction of the higher centers was to transform a sensation of ordinary touch into an experience of acute pain.[6] This observation has since been experimentally confirmed in physiological laboratories.

The importance of these studies for the correct understanding of Janet's concept of equilibrium is very great. At any given moment of our lives, waking or sleeping, we are not in receipt of and responding to merely one or a few sensations. On the contrary, we are continuously in receipt of a mass of sensations, the mass varying not only with the receptors but also with the condition imposed upon the receptors by the nervous system. Some of these sensations pass quickly—in Adrian's term they are "phasic"; others last longer and are "postural."[7] Because of these "numerous inpouring currents of sensation," William James in a much quoted passage described the consciousness of a baby as "one big blooming buzzing confusion." As a comment on this, the author of *Confessio Medici* wrote: "If that was my consciousness once, then glory be to Psyche for making it what it is now." The claim made by James is in one sense good, although his description of the baby's consciousness is almost certainly incorrect. The claim is good in the sense that an infant's

[6]Henry Head, *Studies in Neurology* (London: Oxford University Press, 1920), I, 163.

[7]E. D. Adrian, *The Basis of Sensation* (New York: W. W. Norton & Company, Inc., 1928), p. 79.

receptors are actively in operation; it is bad in that from the first, under the guidance of what is termed instinct, there is selection and order, provided the integrity of response is undamaged. The alternative to integral response is not buzzing confusion but coma.

Provided the integrity of response is undamaged, this phrase covers many types of contributory activity. If, for example, a lecturer addressing an audience is suddenly stunned by someone with a club, he stops speaking; but in addition to this he falls to the ground, and on recovery he may be actively nauseated. If he—the lecturer—is then asked what he was doing, he will undoubtedly reply that he was lecturing; he will not think it necessary to specify, nor can he specify completely, all those other multitudinous activities without the support of which his major action could not have been accomplished. The descriptive sentence above names three types of activities: in inverse order, *reflex, habitual skill, attentive effort.*[8] Janet's claim is that attentive effort is impossible without the support of reflexes, conditioned reflexes, and acquired habitual skills.

The manner in which numerous reflexes operate in support of a chief activity can be variously illustrated. The best known illustration is the almost automatic accommodation of the pupil of the eye to light. Another illustration is the transfer of blood from muscles to liver during digestion, or the transfer

---

[8]For further discussion, see Chapter VI.

of blood to the musculature during active exercise. The possibility of illustration is endless; but the point to observe is that these contributory activities are contrived without the knowledge of the subject, who is completely unaware of what is happening. Such activities are symptomatic of a good heredity and good health. It would be mistaken to suppose, however, that such reflex activities do not change as the organism develops its capacity for response to the world about it. The animal does not directly know, and cannot directly know, what is happening.

Yet it is clear, in higher animals especially so, that reflexes are under control. . . In other words, the reactions of reflex-arcs are controllable by [higher center] mechanisms to whose activity consciousness is adjunct. By these higher centres, this or that reflex can be checked, or released, or modified in its reaction with such variety and seeming independence of external stimuli that the existence of a spontaneous internal process expressed as "will" is the naive inference drawn. . . No exposition of the integrative action of the nervous system is complete, even in outline, if this control is left without consideration. Reflexes ordinarily outside its pale can by training be brought within it.[9]

The manner in which this control of *conditioned reflexes* is contrived is best illustrated by the famous experiments of Pavlov. Pavlov was dealing experimentally with a true reflex, involving the application of meat to a dog's tongue as stimulus and the flow of saliva as response. The experimental advantage was that the reflex response could be measured in drops

[9]Sherrington, *The Integrative Action of the Nervous System,* pp. 388-389.

of saliva, and timed. The dog is never directly aware of, or directly in control of, the salivary response; he is aware of the appearance and taste of the meat and of his own swallowing movements. To succeed in his experiments, Pavlov had to create a highly artificial surrounding: a soundproof and isolated room for the experimental dog (the experimenter being absent) with the ticking of the metronome (or other experimental "condition") being as far as possible the sole variable, apart from the direct stimulus, in the situation. Had he not contrived the situation thus, a sufficient primacy would not have automatically attached itself to the beats of the metronome, or other experimental device. Having contrived his experiment thus, Pavlov found that a dog conditioned to expectation of food with 111 beats of the metronome would salivate to this stimulus but not to 98 or 105 beats. This in an animal that cannot possibly count to one hundred is astonishing evidence of the manner in which reflexes may be syncretistically but exactly conditioned in support of a dominant activity. It is a fair inference from Pavlov's statements, as it is from Sherrington's, that the "conditioning" of reflexes is part of a process of habit organization. Pavlov remarks that, although the control of salivation is exercised by the vegetative nervous system and is subcortical, the experiments do not succeed except in the case of dogs with undamaged cortices; that is, with undamaged capacity for integral response.

The control exercised by an *habitual skill* is an-

E

other matter; it is cortical, it is accompanied by what we call consciousness. There is much physiological work, for example that of Loeb and Lashley, which shows that instinctive response and habit are developed and controlled by the cortex. These two—the earliest congenital responses and the individually acquired aggregates of response—are the basis of all so-called mental activity. It is at this level of activity only that learning, in the strict sense, takes place.

The word *learning* implies the improvement of response to an external object and situation (not to a stimulus merely); it is accompanied by clear awareness of what is happening; the activity is directed outwards and to the improvement of the organism's relation with its surrounding. The chief character of the changed response is its *complication*. G. F. Stout speaks of "the cumulative effect of attention on its own process."[10] The infant, for example, progressively develops a greater complexity of relationship with things and people in the world about it. At one time the difficult business of learning to walk will take immense effort and much practice. Walking later is merely subsidiary to a host of other activities—but still a necessary part of them. Speech also is preceded by the discovery that certain sounds will attract the attention of the important adults that rule the infants' world and will to some extent direct their attention. The understanding of sentences develops some time

---

[10]*A Manual of Psychology* (3d ed.; London: University Tutorial Press, Ltd., 1913), pp. 177 ff.

before the capacity to construct and utter sentences. This general chàracter, that of complication, continues throughout life; it is for every individual the fundamental condition of continued interest in living. Direction of development differs, of course, in different people. The student of walking may become renowned for capacities for running, throwing, and sliding into base. The tyro in speech may become a politician. But in all of us a certain proportionate and basic development of such capacities is necessary to normal living. Walking, speech, motor skills, social understanding are not only differently complicated in different individuals, in any one person the relative importance of this or that element changes as he becomes adult or grows older. Civilization obviously offers multitudinous and various opportunities of different development as compared with any primitive way of living.

Skill thus acquired is exceedingly complex. The complexity of control is most easily illustrated by selecting as an instance something external to the individual exercising that skill. Some of you may have seen the control board of a fighting plane, which is operated by one young man. To those of us whose motor skills have diminished with the years, a moment's inspection of the multiplicity of instruments makes it seem almost impossible that any one individual could attain the necessary unity and perfection of control over a machine that flies at four hundred miles an hour at many heights and in many positions, that is in radio communication with other planes and the military base, that has eight guns to be fired at the appropriate moment, and demands a selection among the projectiles used—first, armour piercing; second, tracer; third, explosive. It is an amazing tribute to the capacity for motor complication of the young pilots that many of them attain an almost perfect unity of operation with their machines. In naming these few items in the complex control I have not even begun to make an exhaustive list of the different contributory activities.

Now skill must make of any such operation a single complex activity, or it is not skill but bungling incompetence. It must include not only capacity to handle external objects but also skill in muscular exertion. An outstanding character of the athlete is that he accomplishes his task with a smaller actual expenditure of muscular energy than an untrained person. "The increased metabolism resulting from muscular exercise is met effectively only in the trained subject, through the coordination of a number of factors, the response, in general, being about what might be expected in a well-integrated system accustomed to such demands."[11] I have vivid recollections of the struggles of an elderly man to learn golf, a man whose previous life had given him only minor mus-

---

[11]A. V. Bock, D. B. Dill, and others, "Studies in Muscular Activity," Part III, "Dynamical Changes Occurring in Man at Work," *The Journal of Physiology,* vol. LXVI, no. 2 (October 10, 1928), p. 159.

cular skills. He was at once the amusement and the despair of his coach. His muscular system had apparently never acquired a capacity for relaxing all muscles other than those in actual use. He took his stance with every muscle cramped and rigid; he gave spectators the impression that he was attempting to hit the ball with both feet off the ground. His long effort to learn was not crowned with success.

These complicated skills—and all skills are complicated—are acquired by patient attention to detail. Practice makes perfect, not because of mere repetition, but because "awkwardness, error and roundabout ways"[12] are not repeated; they are eliminated. Habit is not repetition, although it is commonly described, even by psychologists, as if it were: it is an acquired integral response to a many-faceted situation. And with every exercise it is changed in some particular. The method of change is by means of the process that psychologists call attention, or concentration. This does not mean that in the process of attending to some detail we cease to be aware of its wider context. On the contrary, skilled response to a situation implies an active awareness of the whole context, a readiness immediately to move attention and action from one point to another. The actions occur as a series, but the sequence is dictated by the entire situation; the various actions never, except perhaps in the tyro, succeed one another in a

---

[12]Sir William Mitchell, *The Structure and Growth of the Mind* (London: Macmillan and Co., Limited, 1907), p. 87.

predetermined fashion. Every reader has become directly acquainted with this fact as he drives his automobile through the streets. The greater the actual skill the less are the serial acts predetermined.

Such skill must be acquired in orderly fashion; any complex skill is only gradually developed. The control board of a training plane is much simpler than that of the fighting plane. Moreover, the instruments upon it are all related to the control of a plane in flight. This is already a sufficiently complicated skill to acquire, and the pilot in training is expected to develop adequate and habitual ability in this respect before he is introduced to the further complications involved in fighting as well as flying. The mere act of a given moment may, it is true, be regarded as narrow or narrowly concentrated at a given point. But if the person acting is skilled, the act itself is, as it were, surrounded by a vivid awareness of context directly relevant to what he is doing. If anything occurs that demands attention, it receives it immediately: the attention of a skilled driver who is enjoying the sights and sounds of rural summer will be immediately diverted to his car if one slight sound heralds the possible approach of engine trouble. A less skilled person will not even notice the sound.

A vivid awareness of context is the primary condition of effective attention. The skilled person ignores what is not immediately relevant to action, not because it is meaningless, but rather because it is in fact fulfilling the meaning he is actively assigning it.

At the present moment the reader is either attentive to this chapter or the chapter is conducive to relaxation or thought of tomorrow's activities. The reader is nevertheless actively aware that the room in which he reads has windows, and for so long as they behave as mere windows he will not regard them with special interest or curiosity. But if, for example, a giraffe were suddenly to intrude its head through one of them, the effect would be instantaneous and startling. Every activity—reading, or thought of next day's occupations—would be interrupted; he would turn to inspect the astonishing phenomenon. This, because the appearance of a giraffe is not ordinarily included in the background of the room in which he reads. In other words, the window would have ceased to carry the function he implicitly assigns to it. It is because we do actively assign meaning to the items of a context that they do not attract our attention. It is not because we are unaware or unconscious of them.

This has no doubt seemed a long excursion from Janet's investigations of hysteria. It has been necessary in order to show not only that his equilibrium hypothesis is interesting but that it possesses a descriptive excellence not to be found in any other theory of the nature of psychological development. It is because of the adequacy of this clinical approach that Janet is so good an observer of the exact mental situation of this patient *now*, while under direct observation. I am not claiming that Janet knows best how to deal with such situations therapeutically. On the contrary, he is notably less interested in therapy than in accurate observation. But if one desires to know approximately the mental situation of an hysteric, or the typical defects in an obsessive's method of thinking, the observations of Janet cannot be neglected. He has provided a conceptual scheme or pattern to which skilled observation can be related. This scheme may be briefly expressed thus:

I. Every mental state is an exceedingly complex unity. It is made up of a multiplicity of factors so numerous that psychology cannot completely describe any given instance. Nevertheless these multiple factors in balanced relationship are at any active waking moment arranged in a certain order:

A. *Conditioned Reflexes (control subcortical).*
Reflexes—primary automatisms. These are to some extent "conditioned" by the general developmental process.[13]

B. *Acquired Skills (control cortical).*
Habitual skills—secondary automatisms. These include capacity to give meaning to a situation at a glance, and to respond to it. The result of learning and ac-

---

[13]I. P. Pavlov, *Conditioned Reflexes,* translated and edited by G. V. Anrep (London: Oxford University Press, 1927); Sherrington, *The Integrative Action of the Nervous System.*

quired skill, these capacities constantly undergo alteration by:

C. *The Active Response (control cortical).* The act of attention of a given moment. The point of adaptation or learning.

II. Janet claims that attention, or capacity to respond actively at a given point, is the function of an ordered equilibrium between the above-named multiple capacities. Conversely, the order approximately described above is imposed upon the whole by the active effort of a present moment. Any disequilibrium shows itself immediately in diminished capacity for active function, for alert attention to surrounding. The occasion may be injury, illness, or such interferences as personal disappointment or grief.[14]

It is difficult to see why some of Janet's critics should have discarded as meaningless his concept of psychological tension. He explains the descriptive meaning of this phrase in many of his studies.[15] It is, however, proper in this place to point out that the concept is a legitimate extension of the physiological and neurological studies we have been considering. Bock and Dill[16] speak of the increased metabolism

---

[14]See also Chapter VI.

[15]*Les Obsessions et la Psychasthénie* (Paris: Librairie Felix Alcan, 1919), pp. 453-609; *Les Névroses,* pp. 362-365.

[16]Bock, Dill, and others, "Dynamical Changes Occurring in Man at Work."

resulting from muscular exercise as a product of the coordination of a number of factors in a well-integrated system. When the activity studied is one that involves muscular effort, it is comparatively easy to detect and measure the extra fuel consumption. The fact that the nervous metabolism is not at present readily measurable by existing laboratory methods does not mean that physiology and psychology must instantly dispense with the concept of tension. On the contrary, it is more than ever necessary that physiology should retain a conceptual scheme that has proved so fruitful of results. Indeed, it is only certain psychologists who make an initial assumption that attention is the unit upon which psychological elaborations are based—it is only these psychologists who find themselves unable to understand the necessity and usefulness of Janet's concept for adequate clinical observation. In the sense in which Janet means it, any act of attention is unquestionably the product of a complex equilibrium responding actively at a given point. His description has the further merit of applicability to the responses of an amoeba or a Unio, just as to those of a dog or a human, allowance being made for natural limitations of capacity to complicate at different organismic levels.

One other comment, and this somewhat technical chapter will be ended. I have spoken of our endowment of reflex capacities as the legacy of good heredity and health. This endowment includes not only response but also that to which we respond. In other words, the mass of sensations (of form, color, weight, "togetherness" in a visual field, and so on) into which we later read the significance of a physical and social world are as much conferred upon us by our organism as reflexes and instinctive capacity for development. It is accordingly necessary that, just as we distinguish between subcortical reflex and cortically developed skill, so also must we distinguish technically between the primitive awareness of the sensory mass and the derived meanings we learn to assign to this mass. In one sense, the sensations never change throughout our lives; the *meanings assigned them change* from day to day—indeed, from moment to moment. And the whole mass is perpetually present to us, waking or sleeping; what difference exists is in the activity of response, the momentary assignment of meaning.

One is compelled to admit the possibility therefore of mental disabilities that are related predominantly either to the primitive awareness or to the systems of skilled response. In this respect hysteria would seem to be the mental reflection of a primary and probably organic rift in the sensory mass; in the findings of both Janet and Freud, obsession is on the contrary a disability of response. In so far as this distinction proves to be legitimate, it makes probable a diagnosis of hysteria as a physical malady. This would leave obsessive ills as the proper subject of psychopathological study in the strict sense.

IV

OBSESSIVE THINKING

Janet's researches began with the inquiry into hysteria; there is no description of the actual situation of the somnambule that can equal or rival his. But like all clinicians he was compelled to recognize the existence of another mental disability of a mild type that has nothing in common with hysteria. This is the ill he terms *obsession* or *psychasthenia*. At the time when he began his medical investigation these cases were considered extremely difficult. Obsessive patients were not only proof against all attempts at hypnosis, they tended also to meet well-intended suggestion with prolonged and apparently pointless reasoning and argument. This symptom was frequently resented by physicians and led many of them to believe mistakenly that obsession was a more serious ill than hysteria.

It is a curious fact, indicated by Janet in recent years, that in the modern world the incidence of hysteria, in the strict sense, has notably diminished.

Many of the so-called "shell-shock" cases in the war of 1914-1918 must be excepted from this statement, but, allowing this exception, it may be said that hospitals nowadays can only rarely show a typical somnambule of the Charcot-Janet type. This has not occurred as a consequence of medical advance in diagnosis and therapy, but independently of it. It may be due, at least in part, to a general improvement of nutrition during childhood and to better facilities for education. Freud observed this same fact on his return to Vienna from France; hypnosis was of small practical use to him either as an empirical therapy or as a method of investigation.[1] Many medical officers made a similar discovery when they returned to civilian practice after the last war; they found that the methods used in military hospitals—"shell-shock" cases were often, though not always, hysterics—were of little or no advantage to their civilian patients. In 1922 one such officer told me of a postwar paper he had read to his medical association with actual military case examples of the production and removal of symptoms by hypnosis. His paper ended with a claim that the war had shown physicians how to handle nervous patients and that these methods could be applied in ordinary practice. Somewhat ruefully he admitted that in a subsequent period of six months' work he had not succeeded in hypnotizing one civil-

---

[1]Sigmund Freud, *Selected Papers on Hysteria and Other Psychoneuroses;* also his *Autobiography,* translated by James Strachey (New York: W. W. Norton & Company, Inc., 1935).

ian patient. This physician, like the majority of his colleagues, believed that as the incidence of hysteria diminishes, the incidence of obsession rises. This contention may well possess some validity, but it does not seem possible at present to demonstrate the suspected increase of obsession and anxiety states as evidently as the diminution of hysteria.

Janet's study of obsession was first published in 1903, and even then he had noticed that this type of patient is encountered more frequently in private practice than in public hospitals. He relates this directly to the fact that "a certain measure of intellectual culture plays a part in the development"[2] of obsession. His study is based upon his experience of 325 cases; of these he selects five for special report and groups his observation of the other patients about them. He remarks that the incidence of obsessive thinking is highest between the ages of twenty and forty. His first case, Claire, was a young girl of twenty-eight; she had been studied and treated by Janet for nine years. In this time her condition had improved. The second, Lise, a woman of thirty, had been studied uninterruptedly for five years; at first she was seriously ill but little by little she became better. She was intelligent, educated, and capable of keen observation. The third, John, was thirty-one; he suffered from a mixed condition of overscrupulosity and hypochondria. After only one year with

---

[2]Pierre Janet, *Les Obsessions et la Psychasthénie,* introduction, p. xiii.

Janet, his condition had not notably improved. The fourth, Nadia, was twenty-eight and had been studied for six years. She and the fifth, Gisèle, thirty, had both developed considerable insight into their condition.

Several of the general observations made by Janet call for mention, in order that we shall not forget them when they reappear in the work of the investigators who followed him. The first to be noted is his finding that the incidence of obsession is highest between the ages of twenty and forty. The second is that a certain measure of intelligence and education characterizes those who develop this disability. The third is a comment as to the length of time that is required for the thorough reconstitution of the obsessive's habits of thinking and living. This last shows how widely removed obsessive troubles are from hysteria. The removal of a symptom in an hysterical patient frequently takes no more time than is required for the customary procedure of suggestion. Milne Bramwell records of one of his cases that he could, when requested to do so, send her a post card which instructed her on receipt of the card to sit comfortably somewhere, go to sleep (that is to say, into hypnosis), and after some minutes wake again to find that the objectionable symptom had vanished. There is no possibility of confusing this type of routine procedure with the long re-education required for the identification and control of the closely contrived rationalizations of obsession.

One other comment before proceeding to more detailed consideration of Janet's investigations. At the time when Janet and Freud had respectively embarked upon their interesting researches, the primary assumption for both was necessarily that the inquiry was medical. Perhaps for this reason, we find that neither of them ever quite rid himself of the notion that the ultimate source of these varied mental disorders was organic and possibly pathological. I believe that this assumption has proved itself probable with respect to hysteria; I believe also that the implication of both the Janet and Freud investigations is that many obsessive troubles trace themselves to defects of education in the broadest sense of that term.[3]

The best summary account of Janet's researches is to be found in his small book, *Les Névroses*. Throughout this study he presents in comparative fashion, and alternately, the conclusions of his three larger works on hysteria (*L'Automatisme Psychologique*; *L'État Mental des Hystériques*; *Névroses et Idées Fixes*, vols. I and II) and one on obsession (*Les Obsessions et la Psychasthénie*). He begins his description of obsession by remarking that even the physical appearance, and certainly the manner, of obsessive patients lead the physician immediately to realize that their troubles are very unlike hysteria. He points out that the hysterical patient has usually an amnesia for the speech and action determined by

---

[3]For further discussion, see Chapter VI.

his dissociated secondary self. In his normal condition the hysteric can only report what other persons have told him, namely, that during his so-called "attacks" he is accustomed to speak and act in another manner. Most usually he is incapable of anything in the nature of direct report, except in hypnosis, if he is a true somnambule. He is compelled to rely on the evidence of witnesses. Furthermore, he tends when normal to display a characteristic indifference to topics that excite him profoundly in his alternate condition. Janet's case, Irène, provides a perfect illustration of this.[4]

The obsessive, says Janet, is completely different: "He is embarrassed, uncomfortable, he has trouble in expressing himself; but in reality he knows perfectly what it is that torments him. In place of discovering from the entourage of the patient the subject of his obsessive ideas, it is from the patient himself that we learn the content of the obsession, for he can clearly specify all its details. From this follows the fact that the obsessive crises in which the preoccupation is developed are much less clear-cut than hysterical attacks; obsessive crises have no defined beginning, no definite end. The morbid preoccupation is practically continuous and only at certain moments presents an aspect of active exasperation."[5]

It is from what the patient says that his physician learns what is troubling him, and Janet accordingly

---

[4]*Les Névroses*, pp. 6-8, 12.
[5]*Ibid.*, pp. 16, 17.

attempts an approximate classification of the usual topics of obsessive thinking. He is nevertheless driven to distinguish between the actual topic and the implications of such preoccupation. The actual topic is a much dreaded but continual preoccupation of which the patient can by no means rid himself—a man of forty is horrified to find the thought of a much loved relative recently dead continuously confused with thoughts of defecation—this is obsession.[6] Another patient, a young woman, feels herself driven to acts of horrifying sacrilege—this is compulsion (*"impulsion"*—Janet). The greater number of these patients are shocked to discover in themselves what they believe to be urges to sacrilege, to crime, to sexual irregularity. Janet remarks that it would be amusing if it were not tragic that the majority of the irregularities thus contemplated are not only fantastic but also impossible of actual accomplishment.

In this connection also, as a skilled clinician, he makes a comment which many naive psychoanalysts —I am not referring to Freud—would do well to bear in mind. Many of these patients, he says, men or women, claim to be afflicted with sexual inversion and deplore the sad preference which urges them toward the same sex. Putting aside "the delicate problem of inversion," Janet points out that many of these cases are simply manifesting a common symptom of obsession—the dread that they are possessed by a compulsion to crime or other irregularity. The presence of

---

[6]*Ibid.*, p. 18.

such a symptom should not be too easily accepted as evidence of actual inversion.

The immediate implication of these obsessions is described by Janet as "une honte de soi,"[7] a characteristic self-disgust. It is difficult, he says, to contrive a single word or phrase that will resume and express this attitude. It shows not merely as remorse but as a species of contempt for the subject's own mental attitudes and actions. Religious writers have used the expression "conviction of sin" to describe this; Freud speaks of "conviction of guilt" as an invariable character of the mental background of obsessive thinking. The patient is continuously possessed by the idea that what he is, and what he does, is thoroughly worthless. Everything he does gives rise to self-torment and self-accusation; even when he is not compelled to self-punishment and self-torture, he will decry his own motives and humiliate himself. "Such patients are obsessed by the thought of madness, claim that they are insane, and, what is worse, feel themselves urged to behave as if they were."[8]

These are extreme instances that Janet is describing; he realizes fully that there are many milder cases (which he describes as benign) by comparison with these. But the difference is not to be described simply as between a serious and a mild illness; the symptoms are identical in both instances and the important question seems to be how great an area of

----

[7]*Ibid.*, p. 20.
[8]*Ibid.*, p. 21.

the patient's thinking is affected. This cannot be predicted at the outset; it is only discovered as the investigation proceeds. During the last war I was accompanying a group of medical officers on their rounds in a military hospital for those who were convalescing from nervous troubles. On the outskirts of the group in one ward I noticed a patient suffering from an extreme "forced agitation," obviously anxious to attract the attention of the chief medical officer. Since he was a private soldier and under military discipline, there was no way in which he could do this in summary fashion. I dropped out of the group and talked with him for some time and, when he had sufficiently expressed himself, arranged for his transfer to the headquarters hospital. The next day at headquarters he gave us in great detail the history of the gradual development of his chief symptom—an incessant and distressing micturition. After this one interview, of several hours' duration, he made a rapid and complete recovery. This sounds very like the suggestibility of an hysteric; but in fact, it was nothing of the kind. I must reserve further discussion of this case for a moment; it will then serve to aid the establishment of a distinction between simple and highly complicated obsessive situations. But in the meantime, the abbreviated history will illustrate two observations upon which Janet insists.

The first of these is that the symptom of which the patient complains is not a fragment dissociated from the rest of the subject's mental awareness, as in hysteria. On the contrary, the obsessive pre-occupation is a carefully contrived structure to which the thinking of the individual has day by day contributed this or that element. This has been effected in large part by close and careful reasoning, and in order to justify his particular obsession. In Janet's phrase, there is in such situations "a collaboration of the whole personality,"[8a] a characteristic which is never found in hysteria. There is no automatic incidence of the seeming physical disability— in the instance quoted above, frequent and distressing micturition— without the patient's knowledge as in hysteria, or by reason of some organic unbalance or pathology as in actual illness.[9] The symptom arrives as the inevitable end-product of continuous and highly articulate thinking developed over a period of years. Frequently this thinking has never been expressed in its articulate detail to anyone before the clinical interview. During the interview with an obsessive there is no alternation of mental states or personalities as in hysteria; even if the patient has complained of amnesias, of defective memory, all trace of such limitation vanishes when he begins to talk freely.[10] The patient is perfectly well aware of the reason why, in his estimation, he should suffer such a symptom. Moreover, the conviction of sin enters into the situation as a determinant. The excessive precautions a hypochondriac takes are not primarily intended to ward off externally determined accidents; they are always

---

[8a]*Ibid.*, p. 35.   [9]*Ibid.*, p. 35.   [10]*Ibid.*, p. 48.

designed to protect him against the consequences of his own acts.[11] His bitter conviction of his own worthlessness lies in the immediate hinterland of all his reasoning. But however fantastic in its entirety, his reasoning is continuous and articulate in respect of detail. It is not often possible to select any one item and to brand it as impossible, although the whole structure of his thought may be entirely so. A colleague on one occasion undertook to interview a student, mildly obsessive, who complained of inability to sustain his attention. The interview lasted for six hours, with one interruption for a meal, and during the whole of that time the young man talked without effort, sustained his attention easily and presented a lucid and systematic account of his history and pre-occupations. So also with the military case above mentioned; the talk of several hours' duration consisted of a lucid presentation of the thought structure organized over many years, which had finally issued in the compulsion to micturition. The whole personality of the obsessive individual is actively participant in the symptom determination.

Janets' other observation is to the same effect with respect to what he calls *forced agitation.* The agitation of an obsessive crisis is quite unlike any symptom of hysteria. It is true here as in the obsession itself that the patient is forcing it upon himself by the active participation of his whole intellectual and emotional

---

[11]Janet, *Les Obsessions et la Psychasthénie*, p. 63.

capacity in the crisis. The situation is an exaggeration of the normal; the suspense and anxiety any one of us might feel in awaiting either a report upon a surgical operation or the issue of an aerial combat is here reproduced in an excessive manner. But whereas in the normal situation there are good grounds and external justification for the anxiety, in the obsessive the determinant is the inner reasoning and emotional preoccupation of the individual. Frequently, as in the military case or that of the obsessive student, a considerable part of the forced agitation may disappear, at least temporarily, during a clinical interview.

These two observations call for a comment in passing. In these days many hospital cases are classified as hysteria which bear few, if any, of the stigmata of the typical somnambule. Such patients are usually persons of small education and opportunity who complain of pain or other physical disability that cannot be traced to organic disorder by physician or neurologist. This use of the word hysteria owes allegiance to Freud's suggestion that in hysteria a mental disability is converted into an organic symptom by the patient's "unconscious"; it does not relate itself to Janet's investigations. The hospital patients of whom I speak are not hypnotizable and present none of the characters of dissociation. Furthermore, they show, to the limit of their capacity, the tendency to assume a personal responsibility for the whole of their daily thought and action that is typical of the obsessive patients Janet describes. That is to say, it can be demonstrated that the whole person is somehow participant in the determination of the symptom protested. Dr. J. H. Pratt's class in mental control for certain patients of the Boston Dispensary has illustrated the extent to which such individuals may be helped to health by a careful redetermination of personal attitude. It would seem that obsessive thinking in a less intelligent and less educated person cannot develop the continuous and highly articulate character that it attains in his more intelligent and better educated brother. At a certain point, therefore, the sustained preoccupation breaks down but the misery continues; the consequent forced agitation takes form as pain or other organic symptom. If such a description is approximately correct, the disability is of an obsessive rather than an hysterical type.

This seeming divagation illustrates further the defect in the obsessive method of thinking that Janet is trying to make plain. He calls obsessive patients "the scrupulous"; they seem to be actuated by an exaggerated sense of overresponsibility for all they think and do. They drive themselves to consider and decide upon every minor thought and act as if a moral decision of immense importance were involved. Although they develop their own unhappy compulsive rituals they carefully guard themselves against the acquisition of ordinary habitual routines. Culpin and Smith say of them that they give the impression of always taking the line of greatest resistance.[12] This is the reason why elsewhere I have said, "They are experts in an arduous re-thinking of the obvious—they substitute an exaggerated precision in minor activities for that activity in major affairs of which they are, or feel themselves to be, incapable."[13] This curious refusal to develop the secondary automatisms of habit bores them, makes them utterly miserable and leads in certain instances to profound depression.

The burden of decision is the burden of possible sin; they consequently suffer agonies of indecision. An obsessive soldier when asked if he would like to remove to another hospital remained rigid and unsleeping because he could not decide; in the morning he asked the military doctor to decide for him. It is after these agonies of indecision, characterized by an interminable and inconclusive rehearsal of all the pro and contra arguments to the last pin point of possible difference—it is after these agonies that the characteristic mental exhaustion supervenes. This same individual when he went out for a walk used to "let his feet decide" which path he should take. Janet cites a case entirely similar, a patient who could not act by himself but could do anything otherwise impossible to him if his physician took the respon-

---

[12]Great Britain Industrial Health Research Board, Report No. 61, *The Nervous Temperament,* by Millais Culpin and May Smith (London: H.M. Stationery Office. 1930), p. 10.

[13]Elton Mayo, *The Human Problems of an Industrial Civilization* (2d ed.; Boston: Harvard University, Graduate School of Business Administration, Division of Research, 1946), p. 112.

sibility of ordering it. This same patient could occasionally perform an action habitually difficult if he assured himself: "It is not I who act, it is my hands."[14]

The essential character of the interminable and inconclusive argument is that the question considered lies between false alternatives. Obsessives have a passion for generalization, for false dichotomy; Janet's descriptive phrase is "la manie du tout ou rien."[15] The passion for fine logical distinctions runs into absurdity. A man of forty consulted a physician by reason of extreme obsessive disability; his history showed that he had never contrived to adapt himself to easy association with his fellows—men and women. So far as women were concerned he had a series of reflections which horrified him. In interview he revealed a classification of all women in two contrasting classes —the thin and virtuous, the fat and vicious. He felt that he should marry, and the idea of marriage to any but a thin and virtuous woman was inconceivable. Nevertheless he was attracted only by fat women, and his few would-be virtuous approaches to thin women had been signally unsuccessful. The alternatives he proposed to himself were fantastic and utterly without warrant in the world of fact. But the endless internal argument that exhausted him was conducted entirely in these terms. For many years his intimate thinking on this important human rela-

14*Les Névroses*, p. 168.
15*Ibid.*, p. 54.

tion had been of this general character. His professional work included the teaching of philosophy to adolescents.

This type of thinking becomes accentuated in a crisis until it becomes a "bavardage interieur," an internal chatter, which may easily seem to be entirely meaningless at the beginning of an interview. Nevertheless, if the patient is permitted to talk freely to his physician, after a period of some hours the pattern begins to reveal itself. John, a patient of Janet's used to beseech him "simply to listen" in order to comfort him.[16] And for a period of an hour and a half or two hours he would pour forth a stream of apparently random associations without stopping for a moment. At the end of such a session he confessed himself comforted and relaxed—"he had exhausted in words an agitation of which he could not otherwise rid himself."

It is inevitable that mental habits of this kind should issue in doubt. Undecided, full of doubts, the unhappy obsessive feels that he lives in an unreal world; he feels that he is incomplete, that he lives as a machine doing and saying things without significance. He feels also that the people about him are equally unreal. Nevertheless, he is quite ready to declare his obsessions ridiculous.[17] Here again is illustrated the curious overawareness of his every thought and act that characterizes the obsessive. I was once

[16]*Ibid.*, p. 79.
[17]*Ibid.*, p. 49.

asked by the leading physician of a medical group to interview one of his younger colleagues who, he said, was suffering "a distressing anxiety condition." I found that the wife of the young man was also a medical practitioner. She met me at the door and took me to her husband's room. He was in bed, restless, a large book open beside him. By way of beginning a conversation I remarked that he hadn't got up and asked why. He stopped tossing on the bed and replied, "Because I was afraid I might be hit by a meteorite." This was not a very good beginning, nor did it sound exactly like obsession; so I tried again. Looking at the book, I said, "What is it you are reading?" "The British Encyclopaedia," he said, "the section on meteorites." I asked if he had got any comfort from it. "At the beginning," he replied, "it says that when meteorites reach the earth's atmosphere they usually dissipate into dust." "You didn't get up," I said. "No," he replied, "a little further down it says that sometimes they don't."

From this point on we talked quite easily, and presently he said to me: "I know that what I think is ridiculous, but the trouble is that I cannot help thinking it." He was at the time something over thirty years of age; the preoccupation about meteorites had already established itself when he was four. I shall later explain that the preoccupation was not significant for his disability or in any sense determinant of it. This is frequently the case; the particular dichotomy—in this instance, danger or no danger from falling meteorites—that floats to the surface, as it were, in a first interview is very rarely a significant determinant. I quote his case here merely to show that his mental situation—in a country very far from France—showed the structure Janet describes as typical, an intense preoccupation with false alternatives that cannot be by any means resolved, an exaggerated sense of personal responsibility for its resolution by logical means to the last possible detail, and beyond this a clear knowledge of the absurdity of the antithesis combined with a feeling of personal unreality.

Comparable with this, and indeed issuing from it, is the obsessive's need for "indefinitely recommencing the verification" of this and that.[18] Obsessive preoccupation seems to predispose the individual to the development of elaborate rituals in all the ordinary affairs of living—rituals of hand washing, of putting letters in envelopes, of trying doors a definite number of times to ensure that they are locked. These rituals relate themselves to that arduous re-thinking and re-verification of the obvious of which I have already spoken. Such a method of living clutters the day, and night, with utterly useless elaborations; it makes life miserable for the sufferer and his friends. These futile elaborations are not to be confused with complication in the technical sense—although the habitual complaint of the patient is that he is more complicated than those about him. Normal development takes form as an increasing complication which involves,

---

[18]*Ibid.*, p. 21.

in reality, a greater complexity of relationship with people and things. Obsessive elaboration is not based only upon the oversimplifications of the "tout ou rien" attitude, such false dichotomies as "lean-virtuous" and "fat-vicious" women—it is also an abstract elaboration at this level which actually prevents the obsessive from *complicating* his relationships with other people and condemns him to the barren monotony of repetitive self-centered rituals. Psychoneurotic situations are simpler than normal situations; they are, in fact, insufficiently complex.

V

OBSESSION AND THE
EQUILIBRIUM HYPOTHESIS

Janet's discussion of the many and various symptoms of obsession does not imply that all these symptoms are equally characteristic of every patient. On the contrary, every case is individual and different and must be given the closest clinical study on its own account. Nevertheless, he claims, and with justice, that any adequate description of a particular instance will be found to be capable of statement in terms of an admixture of all or any of the characteristics he has specified. If it be said that case histories which are very like those Janet cites are sometimes the prelude to more serious mental breakdown, the answer is that account must be taken not only of the case history but also of the kind of breakdown when it comes. It is typical of obsession that the so-called "breaks" are crises of agitation and, as such, are no more than a passing intensification of the ordinary condition of the patient. "La préoccupation est presque continuelle et presente simplement des moments d'exaspération."[1] As distinguished from this, Janet points out that in dementia "one finds oneself faced with a chaotic dust heap of ideas, habits, instincts—the dust heaps replacing constructions that have fallen into the completest ruin."[2] It is characteristic of obsession that it is a mental attitude of one-sided overconstruction which is jealously and continuously guarded by the patient. This—the defect of a good quality—cannot be described as bearing any resemblance either to hysteria or to more serious forms of mental breakdown. How then does Janet describe it?

In the first place, he selects two general characteristics of obsessive thinking, the presence of which is always revealed by accurate clinical observation. He calls these "the loss of the function of the real" and "the lowering of psychological tension."[3] As with all clinical description, these phrases mean little in themselves and call for exposition. Both refer to what is essentially the same phenomenon, but, whereas the loss of a sense of reality is direct description of a characteristic symptom, the lowering of psychological tension restates this symptom in terms of Janet's equilibrium hypothesis.

Janet's first point is that the crises of obsessive thinking, the moments when the mental distress is exasperated, relate themselves to some action in the

---

[1]Janet, *Les Névroses*, p. 17.
[2]*Ibid.*, p. 343.
[3]*Ibid.*, pp. 346-367.

present which the patient cannot perform. To the contention that he cannot act because he is afraid, because some phobia prevents him, Janet replies that this is not his opinion at all, that his thesis reverses this claim; in reality, he continues, all the mental distress and agitation is secondary and conceals other and deeper troubles.[4] These other troubles, which are invariable and fundamental, are of the nature of incapacity for adequate and active response to some present situation; the anxieties and distress are derived complications. It is characteristic that the obsessive "has retained all his mental capacities, but has lost the feeling the rest of us always have—rightly or wrongly—that we constitute an actual part of reality, of the present world."[5]

Janet illustrates this aspect of obsessive thinking in various ways. He observes not merely that there is an actual incapacity for adequate action, but that the patient himself is aware of the inadequacy and gives expression to it. The common complaint is of feelings of incompleteness, of a reality that seems dreamlike and further removed from the patient than from other people: many describe themselves as moving and speaking like a mechanical figure that plays a part in some imaginary drama. Any one of us can at once recognize this sympathetically, for we have all had passing experiences of a similar kind in moments of extreme fatigue or when constrained to go

---

[4] *Ibid.*, pp. 161-162.
[5] *Ibid.*, p. 355

G

through the fulfillment of a customary routine in a time of stress or sorrow. At such times we, like the obsessive, feel that we are not wholly participating in the events around us; like him also at such times we tend to read our own diminished participation into the event as a diminished actuality. But whereas with the normal person such a mood passes, with the obsessive it persists. To this Janet traces the frequent use by patients of such adjectives as "unreal," "dreamlike," "strange." To it also he traces the curious experience he describes as the *déja vu,* the feeling many patients have that they have experienced somewhere before in exactly the same manner the events occurring about them. "The essential of the *déja vu,*" says Janet, "is rather the negation of the present than the affirmation of the past."[6]

The mental capacities of the obsessive, he continues, are untroubled in their exercise upon abstract or imaginary objects; symptoms of disorder do not appear until there is some demand for present and concrete activity. The past also, like the imaginary and the abstract, is handled with equivalent ease, but "the present has the effect of an intrusion." The most acute difficulties occur in connection with a need for decision and action in the present. At such a time the characteristic indecisions and doubts, the crises of revery, appear in full force. The only actions obsessives can lightly undertake are those that are insignificant and of small real efficacy. "They can

---

[6]*Ibid.,* p. 356.

walk with, talk with, or complain to, their intimates; but the moment that some action becomes important, they cease to be able to act and, by slow degrees, they abandon their occupation or trade, their external activities, their social relationship—all of which seem, to them, to involve a struggle against other persons."[7]

Action and association (that is to say, easy association with other people)—these are the serious problems. Throughout his studies Janet's observations compel him to insist upon the difficulty of social acts for the victims of obsession. This applies not only to participation in a team effort (a collaboration which they cannot achieve, for they are solitary workers), it may apply also to action in the presence of other people.[8] Indeed, the need to accomplish even the simplest routine before other persons—"to enter an omnibus, to seat herself at table, to write a letter"[9]—such social acts are for his patient "Ger." the occasion of a typical "crisis of revery." Her intense preoccupation with the subject of fasting on Fridays was induced by a simple need to go downstairs to dinner. For these patients every social occasion is an emergency, a crisis that can be met only by the development of immense "drive." And, if the effort is made, the patient afterwards suffers extreme exhaustion.

In another small book[10] Janet says: "Many of these patients are exhausted not by the aftereffect of

---

[7]*Ibid.*, p. 357.   [8]*Ibid.*, p. 165.
[9]*Ibid.*, p. 279.
[10]*La Medécine Psychologique* (Paris: Ernest Flammarion, 1928), p. 254.

some early misadventure but by the present difficulties of a social surrounding too complicated for their mental capacity, which faces them at every moment with a multitude of entangling relationships" that bring their activities to a standstill. After discussing methods by which a wise physician will attempt a simple preliminary "disentanglement" of the patient from the claims which press, or seem to press, upon him, Janet comments: "Psychological analysis shows us clearly that social actions are the most complex human activity and that the costs exacted by adaptation to the individuals around us are by far the heaviest."[11] In his other studies he has demonstrated that timidity and incapacity for social effort are characteristic. He proceeds to trace the downward trend from mere timidity as the mental depression becomes deeper in an individual instance. At first perhaps no more than a fear of strangers and of appearances on public occasions, the general timidity develops more and more in the direction of an inability to live with those who constitute the patient's normal entourage. This finds expression in a desire for solitude which almost always formulates itself in the dream of a "desert island."[12]

This finding has been extensively confirmed by other physicians. It may have been operative in determining the special character of the Weir Mitchell treatment. A medical colleague in Queensland, near-

---

[11]*Les Névroses*, p. 255.
[12]*Ibid.*, p. 256.

ly thirty years ago, found that the first desirable step in treatment of such cases was to isolate them from their immediate relatives, to impose a preliminary simplification of living in exactly the manner Janet recommends. The so-called ambivalence of attitude towards immediate relatives that has been so emphasized by the Freudian school originates no doubt in many instances as Freud describes it. It is, however, to be observed that acute situations of this type are usually a late development and are, at least in part, a manifestation of the mental exhaustion Janet describes. The patient feels that he can no longer keep up with what is expected of him by his immediate circle.

Discussion of Janet's phrase, the "loss of the function of the real," has brought us back by a long detour to an observation made in the first chapter. The reality about all of us is a socio-reality; every routine, every habit involves association and collaboration with other persons. It is to this social aspect of reality that obsessives are almost completely unadapted. Meeting other people, collaborative effort—to those of us who have been fortunately conditioned socially —these things are delightful and do not involve difficulty. It is not so with the obsessive—for him each successive social occasion implies a new emergency. Where the majority of people adapt easily and without any sense of exertion, the obsessive is committed to an exaggerated concentration of attention upon minute details of association. This has the effect of removing him still further from group participation, because his attitude seems too individual and decidedly peculiar to other persons—a fact that he himself perceives with bitter clarity. And it is at this point that he develops not only the dream of a "desert island" but also the feeling of a need to defend himself against this hostile world— "ce monde hostile."[13]

A brief summary of the observations recorded in the first chapter in connection with the six "destroyers" and the "gunman" is directly relevant. These observations were:

1. These men had no friends except at the propagandist level. They seemed incapable of easy relationship with other people; on the contrary, the need to achieve such relation was for them an emergency demanding energetic effort.

2. They had no capacity for conversation. Their talk alternated between self-history and oratory which reproduced the compelling topic—the destruction of society.

3. All action, like social relationship, was for them emergency action. Any idea of routine participation in collaborate effort, or the "ordinary," was conspicuously absent. Everything, no matter how insignificant, was undertaken with immense and unreasoned "drive."

4. They regarded the world as a hostile place.

---

[13]Janet, *Les Obsessions et la Psychasthénie,* p. 636.

Every belief and action implied that society existed not to give but to deny them opportunity. Furthermore, they believed this hostility to be active, not merely inert; they regarded everyone, even their immediate associates, as part of the forces arrayed against them.

These observations may be applied to the elucidation of every obsessive situation; but the immense difference between those who react as the "destroyers" do and those who feel the need for defense and solitude must be reaffirmed. Janet is clearly aware of this difference; he remarks in this connection:

> The problem is that of distinguishing between psychasthenic states which manifest a tendency to evolve towards systematic distortion of attitude (*délires*) and those which are destined to limit themselves to obsession. Previous indications of character—egocentricity, pride, susceptibility, authoritarian ideas—betray an inclination to objectify psychological troubles, to attribute to the machinations of other people the subject's own psychological insufficiencies. Moreover, one finds in this group an increased tendency to systematization and less disposition to obsessive doubt. . . Conversely, sweetness, humility, a tendency to perpetual subjective analysis are indications in a patient of the approach of indecision, doubt, and the typical over-scrupulous attitude.[14]

Janet's estimate of the comparative incidence of these two forms is that the latter type comprises "more than two-thirds" of the total.[15] Experience

---

[14]*Ibid.*, p. 697.
[15]*Ibid.*, p. 636.

elsewhere seems to confirm this estimate. In the first chapter the two attitudes were expressed as "the world is hostile, let me attack it," and "the world is dangerous, I must be very careful." It is the latter, the typically obsessive attitude, which chiefly concerns us; patients of this type objectify their own psychological insufficiency by reading into the world about them a diminished reality.[16] The former type is, in extreme, murderous in attitude to other people; the latter is definitely suicidal, indeed the great majority of those who commit suicide belong unquestionably to the obsessive group.

This can be illustrated by report of an actual suicide. The subject was a student residing in college, whose sudden death came as a surprise to his associates. In a newspaper account of the tragedy he was described as an ardent student of politics and military affairs; he was a hard worker and stood high in the estimate of his teachers. His relations with his immediate family, however, were unhappy; he had shown increasing reluctance to return home for his vacations. Those who knew him best emphasized his loneliness. He had a reputation for being reserved and quiet; it was his custom at meal times to seat himself remotely from other students in dining hall or restaurant. Occasionally when with others he would begin an intense discussion of some political topic and apparently was not easily able to stop even if the moment was obviously inappropriate. He had

---

[16]For further illustrations, see "Frightened People" in the appendix.

been known to express the view that this tendency served to alienate those who might have been his friends: from this derived an accentuated aloofness from others, which did not wholly conceal a deeply rooted conviction of futility and deprivation. Further inquiry showed the newspaper account to be accurate, other details merely extended and intensified the picture of a lonely individual keenly anxious for human friendship but utterly unable to achieve it. And the very defences he had contrived effectively barred him off from those college agencies which nowadays exist to discover and aid such individuals.

Discussion of Janet's observations on the diminished reality of an obsessive life may have seemed to make his other concept of "lowered psychological tension" more difficult. It might be claimed, for example, that this ever-present sense of emergency and the drive to overcome it are evidences of higher rather than lower tension. And indeed if this were an argument about words, or the possible meanings of words, the point might present considerable difficulty. This is not, however, what Janet is considering. His equilibrium hypothesis has shown what is necessary to integrity of response in the daily routines of every individual. The awareness of any given moment is not a simple unit of thought, a simple act of attention. There is, of course, some dominant or attentive activity, but this is no more than the final expression at the point of action of an exceedingly complex unity—an immense multiplicity of factors, both of awareness and of response, in mutually balanced relationship.

This complex equilibrium is found upon investigation to present what Janet calls a hierarchy, an ordered arrangement, of psychological phenomena.[17]   He terms the arrangement hierarchical because the range is from low-level to high-level phenomena. At the lowest level are primary automatisms, reflexes—the legacy of good heredity and health. Just above this are conditioned reflexes as described by Pavlov and Sherrington. Above this again are the special instincts which in their earliest action seem almost identical with reflexes but differ from them in that they are subject to learning, to memory and, in a word, to developed cortical control. Out of these develop the secondary automatisms of habit and skill. Only in situations where the ordered balance between these many and various capacities is in smoothly working order is the final activity, the attention of a given moment, possible. This hypothetical description has the full support of Pavlov, Sherrington, and neurologists generally; it is indeed a carefully contrived extension of the neurological concepts of facilitation, inhibition, and integral response.

It is with this in mind that Janet is able to look back and forth from his patients to this conceptual scheme and to his patients again, and so to make certain observations of profound import and value. The first of these is that to which reference has already been made, namely, the lowered psychological tension of obsessive thinking. And here we have to be

---

[17]*Les Névroses,* p. 361.

wary: ordinarily we assume that if we know the usual meaning of a word we know also what it means in a scientific context. We have said that the obsessive attitude is characterized—especially when faced with the need for action or for social activity—by emergency, crisis, drive. This gives rise to the comment that obsessives are "high-strung" or tense, an assertion which has a similitude of objective validity. Looking more closely at such patients, however, Janet observes that they lack certain of the habitual and acquired skills that are essential to ordinary living.

One sees that such persons lead a quite special existence, perfectly insignificant from any viewpoint—withdrawn from things, withdrawn from everyone. They are not interested in anything practical; sometimes from infancy onwards they have shown a most astonishing clumsiness. The family of such a patient always declares that he has never been practical, that he does not know how to take account of his real situation or how to succeed in anything. When such persons retain any capacity for activity, one observes that it will always be in an area far withdrawn from material reality: sometimes they are psychologists, above all things they love philosophy and become terrible metaphysicians. When one has had much experience with obsessives, one arrives at the point of sadly asking whether philosophical speculation is no more than a malady of the human mind.[18]

In order that action, and especially social action, may be prompt and adequate, it is necessary that a full complexity of relationship with the situation be achieved. If the appropriate habitual, skilled relation-

---

[18]*Ibid.*, p. 357.

ships have not been established, the final act of attention cannot be fully or satisfactorily accomplished. One who drives an automobile cannot, for example, watch the road or the traffic until the actual handling of steering wheel, brake, accelerator, and so on has become a supporting complex of secondary automatic activities. Similarly, one who has never learned to handle a knife and fork is hardly likely to make notable contributions to conversation at the dinner table. Janet is concerned to point out that the tension necessary to adequate performance cannot be achieved if any of the minor contributory activities are missing. He insists that in such situations one will always observe a number of inferior and exaggerated activities (or, if you will, tensions) that are substituted for the main action that cannot be accomplished. But these inferior tensions signal, as it were, the incapacity to achieve that complexity of relationship without which the appropriate response is impossible.

This can be illustrated from experiments in the physiological laboratory. The capacity to perform certain tasks—weight lifting, running a certain distance at a certain pace—may be regarded as the product of capacity to produce a certain measurable tension, measured by performance. The runner of marathons can run farther over a longer distance than others; he produces the tension, the performance, by a better integration of muscular effort, of blood supply and oxygen use, which is, in large part, the result of training, of achieved skills and conditioning. The unskilled runner uses his muscles in comparatively clumsy fashion, suffers oxygen debt, excess lactic acid, and fatigue.[19] The former can achieve the tension necessary to performance; the latter cannot, and suffers distress, breathlessness, and muscular stiffness—these last representing the inferior and exaggerated symptoms of incapacity to accomplish. The application of skill is dependent upon the close organization of numerous contributory capacities. This is what Janet means, in a slightly different context, when he says that psychoneurotic situations are less complex than normal situations—they are, in fact, insufficiently complex. Those symptoms that are commonly indicated by the term "high-strung" are the "inferior and exaggerated operations"[20] which are evidence of incapacity for adequate action.

Intellectualism is such a symptom. This assertion does not apply to intelligent development that extends and reinforces action; it does apply to arid intellectualism that is substituted for executive capacity. "Who would not believe," says Janet, "that syllogistic reasoning does not demand more brain work than the perception of a tree or a flower with full experience of their actuality. Yet I believe that so-called common sense is badly deceived on this point. The most difficult operation, that which disappears most

---

[19]A. V. Bock, D. B. Dill, and others, "Dynamical Changes Occurring in Man at Work," p. 159.   [20]Janet, *Les Névroses*, p. 367.

rapidly and most frequently in all conditions of mental disability or depression, is *the apprehension of reality in all its forms.* Medical investigation has forced upon us the recognition of this important fact."[21] Janet's claim must not be supposed to diminish the importance of intellectual development. What he points out is that if intellectual elaborations are not actively related to performance, to experiment at a given point, then such elaborations do not aid the individual to develop or complicate his relation to his surrounding: on the contrary, they tend to be substituted for it and, temporarily at least, to delay or even put an end to such development. Should this happen in a given instance a downgrade movement begins, the individual increasingly substitutes endless debate for action, his capacity for action diminishes, and terrors begin to manifest themselves. Incidentally, Janet is describing the difference between an experimental science and an arid metaphysic incapable of demonstration or proof.

This is unquestionably the mental situation of many obsessives. Their thinking is not only "over-logicked"—"endless discussions that swing back and forth all night and get nowhere"— but it is dominated by a curious assumption that no action may be undertaken until the logic of such action is completely and finally predetermined. The ideas of experiment or adventure are ruled out—and with the banishment of these ideas the possibility of normal mental growth

---

[21]*Ibid.,* pp. 361-362.

is equally banished. Obsessive notions of social participation are also inadequate. In the earlier stages of recovery, when social development is recommended to such persons, the report of their first endeavors is peculiarly characteristic. Sometimes such a person will appear in the morning and report an evening's effort with glowing satisfaction; and one discovers that in a group of people he has completely dominated all discussion and believes himself to have scored a social success. Or it may be that he will appear with his former mental depression reinstated and assert that a social life is not for him; and one discovers that he has attempted to dominate a discussion, has failed, and has withdrawn from it completely. On such occasions he is apt to fortify his damaged self-esteem by claiming to be an intellectual far removed from the diversions of the vulgar. Any idea of routine participation in collaborate effort, or of "the ordinary" in human association, is conspicuously absent.

THE ADAPTIVE MOMENT

1. Reflexes (and organic processes generally).[1]

2. Conditioned Reflexes.[2]

3. Acquired Skills and Habits:

    a. Direct Experience (*knowledge-of-acquaintance*)[3]

        1) Manipulative and technical skills—Things.

        2) Social skills—People.

    b. Reflective Experience (*knowledge-about*).[4]

        1) Situational and clinical thinking—Syncretistic.[5]

        2) Logical thinking—Abstract.

4. The Point of Attention.

Brace annotations (left margin): HOMEOSTASIS[4] — INTEROFECTIVE (groups 1, 2) — EXTEROFECTIVE (groups 3, 4)

For notes see page 110.

VI

THE PSYCHOLOGY
OF ADAPTATION

The accompanying verbal diagram is designed to present Janet's main doctrine in a summary fashion. It perhaps serves to show how closely related his work is to that of the distinguished neurologists and psychologists to whom reference is made.[6] In all his writings Janet claims many times over that the active attention of any given moment is the end result of an exceedingly complex mental and organic state. The diagram is designed to suggest how complex every such act of attention is. Janet maintains, and rightly, that the best indication or symptom of normality is the ability every physically fit person possesses of turning his attention, immediately and easily, to a topic or object presented for his consideration by his surrounding. If he is ill, obviously his capacity to do this will be immediately affected.

---

[6]The reader may wish to refer to the cases described in the appendix to which the concepts underlying the diagram may be readily applied.

Even a simple headache or a feverish condition of increased bodily temperature will instantly show in a diminution of capacity to give and maintain attention to this or that in his vicinity.

But a condition of organic fitness or unfitness, Janet maintains, is not the only determinant of this capacity. As the individual lives and learns, he develops skills of many and various kinds. An academic lecturer in the classroom depends for effective success as much upon his capacity for correct speech and articulate expression, as much upon his capacity for mere walking or using chalk upon the blackboard, as upon his knowledge of the subject he is discussing. In Chapter III I have said that, if such a person is asked what he is thinking about, he will name only the subject of his immediate attention. But in order that he may be free to give his attention easily and accurately to the topic, he must be able to take for granted an undefined number of these contributory skills.

Janet's discussion of obsessive thinking has a special interest for those of us who are mainly concerned with problems of individual psychology, or of social relationships. A person whose mental condition is obsessive, he shows, is unable to give his attention easily and adequately to any topic offered for his consideration. If the reason for this incapacity is found to be due to the interference of "crises of revery," he is termed *obsessive*;[7] that is to say, his

---

[7] Janet, *Les Névroses*, p. 79.

difficulties are due to the interference of habitual and distressing preoccupations concerning problems that he can neither solve nor dismiss.

And Janet goes on to show that this incapacity in the great majority of instances is due to a failure to develop in infancy and adolescence those social skills that are necessary to the most ordinary human communication with other people.

In *La Medécine Psychologique* he maintains, consequently, that even though some one incident during infancy may be significant for the understanding of an individual failure to develop social skills, nevertheless, the physician must take account of the entire infantile and adolescent history, since only the long-range history will account for the failure to develop the very ordinary capacities for easy human interrelationships that characterize the normal person.[8]

Every moment of our waking lives is an adaptive moment. Continually we discover that some one or other of our customary perceptions or ideas is inadequate. The development of skill therefore demands additional experience and reconsideration of the inadequacy. This moreover affects not only our mental life of active effort, it affects also those moments of relative passivity that we characterize as reflective thinking. The importance of reflection to the development of knowledge and skill was strongly emphasized by Janet in lectures and in conversation. The full importance that he assigned to reflection, as

---

[8]Page 254.

the contrary of suggestibility, is nowhere adequately discussed, at least in those books that I have recommended in these notes. There is some discussion of the topic, however, in *Les Médications Psychologiques.*[9]

It is *by reflection*, Janet says, that *we give unity to our experience.* In moments of reflective thinking, our attention is withdrawn from the outer world, and we are preoccupied with some problem that we may, if asked, find difficult to define. But this at least can be said, that at such moments some recent experience has caused us to doubt the adequacy of one of our conceptual schemes, or systems of ideas that we have been accustomed to use. And at such moments we are, whether we know it clearly or not, occupied with an endeavor to reconcile the contradiction or to decide upon a direction of inquiry that will throw new light on the apparent inconsistency. Reflective thinking, therefore, may be described as an inner act of attention, demanded by experience, intimately concerned with the systematic arrangement or rearrangement of our knowledge. This is what Janet means when he says that it is by reflection that we give unity to our experience.

The person who shows symptoms of obsession is unable to put any finality into his reflective thinking. The conception of experiment, of trial and error, has eluded him; he is attempting to solve all the problems

---

[9]Translated by Eden and Cedar Paul, *Psychological Healing,* I, 273-276.

of living by sheer logic in situations where he has had little or no experience. He is consequently a person who is unable to give unity to his experience. He is preoccupied incessantly with persistent efforts to create a merely logical harmony in his thinking; and his misused reflective powers consequently inhibit his capacity for normal and easy attention to events about him. This incapacity limits the systematization of his responses to things, persons, and actuality. In other words, incessant preoccupation with verbal topics interferes with the development of his capacity to give attention to events. It is not surprising, therefore, that the obsessive lacks social and other skills. In this sense obsessive thinking is an ill of education and is therefore of immense interest to students of sociology and psychology.

But the student of sociology or of industry has more to learn from Janet. So far we have learned: first, that every successful attentive act is dependent upon an immensely complex and systematically ordered background of contributory skills and reflexes; and, second, that the relationship between active attention (or the exercise of skill) and passive (or reflective) thinking is all important. If the interplay between action and reflection-upon-such-action is not mutually complementary, then the thinking of the individual is apt to develop in the direction of obsessive interference with all decision and action.

There is another point to add. So far we have considered Janet's studies of the obsessive from a point of view obviously demanded by clinical work. His patients exhibit the two symptoms described above, namely, an incapacity to make decisions or to act, and, second, an incapacity either to develop reflective thinking or to alternate action and reflection in the normal fashion.

But, and this is important, in *Les Névroses*[10] and elsewhere Janet points out that these symptoms will be reproduced accurately, if not permanently, in any situation where, by reason either of external social constraint or of fatigue, an individual is prevented from following the line of development that his own interest dictates. Especially in situations where such constraint prevents the individual from *complicating* his thinking in the manner such thinking demands, he will begin to display the usual symptoms of irritability, indecision, and loss of interest in his work.[11]

The three simple claims of the Janet psychology that I have here outlined are of extraordinary importance to all students of society. The first two—the complexity of the attentive act and the interrelation of action and reflection—he should study under the guidance of a competent psychologist in preparation for his work. This he must do in order that he shall be able instantly to detect the third group of symptoms—constraint and the emergence of obsessive thinking—when such symptoms appear in any

---

[10]Pages 358 ff.

[11]For an instance of this, see Mayo, *Social Problems of an Industrial Civilization*, p. 29.

social or industrial situation he is studying. For the appearance of such symptoms will warn him that there is some irksome constraint or feeling of insecurity imposed upon the individual or group studied by the general conditions of the surrounding. If the student does not proceed to discover what is the source of this feeling of constraint or insecurity, he will remain unable to understand intelligently the social situation he is studying.

Notes for page 102

[1]Sherrington, *The Integrative Action of the Nervous System;* J. M. Charcot, *Maladies du Système Nerveux* (3d ed.; Paris: V. Adrien Delahaye et Cie, 1877), vols. I. II, and III; W. H. Gaskell, *The Involuntary Nervous System* (New ed.; London and New York: Longmans, Green and Co., 1920); J. N. Langley, "The Sympathetic and Other Related Systems of Nerves," *Text-Book of Physiology,* edited by E. A. Schäfer (London: Young J. Pentland, 1900), II, 616-696; Head, *Studies in Neurology,* vols. I and II; Pavlov, *Conditioned Reflexes;* Walter B. Cannon, *The Wisdom of the Body* (New York: W. W. Norton & Company, Inc., 1932).

[2]Pavlov, *Conditioned Reflexes;* Sherrington, *Integrative Action of the Nervous System;* Cannon, *Wisdom of the Body.*

[3]William James, "The Relations of Minds to Other Things," *The Principles of Psychology,* vol. 1, chapter viii, pp. 199-223.

[4]Cannon, *Wisdom of the Body.*

[5]Jean Piaget, *The Language and Thought of the Child* (New York: Harcourt, Brace & Company, Inc.; London: Kegan Paul, Trench, Trubner & Co., Ltd., 1926).

APPENDIX
FRIGHTENED PEOPLE[1]

I shall begin by limiting my topic in two directions. I have no intention, for example, of quoting cases of a psychiatric type. I hope that such instances as I cite will be nearer the facts. This somewhat ambiguous phrase must not be taken to imply any aspersion upon a modern and most valuable development in medicine. I owe too much to psychiatry and psychiatrists to be guilty of such ingratitude. My meaning is merely that when I cite a case, I hope that it will be immediately possible for every member of the audience instantly to translate it into terms of his own experience—into terms of a similar situation with which he is directly acquainted.

The other limitation is that no question of the organic or mental origin of a disorder will be raised—as if these were alternate possibilities. I have no thesis, overt or implied, that the origin of any ill is "all mental." On the contrary, I assume in every instance an organic disability of some kind—unbalance, infection, defect, pathology: but I assume also the existence of other factors of varying importance. These two limitations make it evident that I am confining my attention to the simple and the obvious.

[1]An address given on January 18, 1938, at the Harvard Medical School. First printed in the *Harvard Medical Alumni Bulletin*, January, 1939.

My comfort in this admission must be that the simple and the obvious are perhaps not often enough or not clearly enough stated.

A patient is a case—a case of something that can be looked up in a medical dictionary (B for botulism, T for typhoid); he is also a human being. Both aspects are important to the physician. In the medical schools of thirty or forty years ago the most elaborate care and attention were given to study of the former, the ailment, in clinic, hospital, and laboratory; no attempt was made to develop any systematic study of the human being. I shall later claim that this neglect was not altogether unjustifiable in the social circumstance of that time. But for the moment I wish merely to point out that the neglect carried curious consequences for the practice of medicine. For example, it was very generally believed in those days that the student who did best in his studies was very rarely the man who did best in professional practice afterwards. I am not interested in the truth or falsity of this belief; its interest here is merely as evidence that in some inarticulate way the physicians of that time were already aware of an omission in their general training.

Now when a patient walks into a consulting room he requires two kinds of aid from the physician. The first is medical attention, the second is assurance: in the ordinary consultation the second is as important as the first. The need of assurance is not adequately met by a hearty manner—nor by dogmatism or breezy self-confidence. The world is less suggestible than it used to be, and more obsessive. Especially in these days of universal education the assurance offered must be discriminating; it must be pointed at a particular item in the particular mental context—an item that has been discovered to be there. This differs in different patients, and is almost always left to the physician to discover. By this I mean that the physician is never told directly what the need is; sometimes, usually indeed, the patient cannot tell him, sometimes he does not want to. But in very many instances the physician's success will depend upon discovery of the exact locus of the need for assurance. The physician must therefore make two diagnoses: one of the organic ill, the other of the need of assurance. The latter is often simple, rather easily discovered. But it is unwise to ignore it because it is simple.

Almost twenty-five years ago in Queensland a young doctor came to me at the University and made a statement to the effect that his patients always suffered a "functional complication"—in the phrase of that time—of an organic ill. His practice, which was large, was in a good residential district and the average case was not very serious. He claimed that in the majority of these instances it was not difficult to mitigate, or to get rid of, the organic condition. "And then I find," he added, "that the patient is no better. I have done nothing to get rid of the functional complication." This young man had taken a very good degree at a famous British university; he was very keenly interested in his work. In addition to this he was a high-minded and sympathetic human being. He had always attempted to make an approach to the person in a consultation. The method he had adopted was to assume in the patient an interest equal to and like his own. He would draw diagrams, take down a textbook, explain the nature of the disorder. And this method had no success at all. His patients had no desire to become amateurs of science or medicine; each one wanted reassurance as a person. The more the doctor enlarged upon "the case," the more the patient felt it as annihilation of the person. The physician was defeating his own admirable intention.

After some discussion he realized his error and determined to change his method. From this time on, he attempted to discover the fear and to reassure. The sequel was interesting: in a few months his practice had greatly increased; in a few years he had given up general medicine and become a specialist.

A person in need of assurance is a frightened person; but it is evident that the nature and degree of the fear will differ in different people. If the assurance is to be of the right kind and addressed to the appropriate locus in every individual instance, then the physician is in need of an approximate classification that will help him to identify, and be sufficiently adequate to, the situation set before him. With this in mind, and for purposes of ordered discussion, I have devised a classification of three types of personal situations. The classification is arbitrary and empirical; it is based upon an approximate estimate of the kind of fear and its distribution in the individual's thinking. In the simpler cases there is not much fear and what there is tends to attach itself to the actual organic disorder. In the more difficult cases there is a great deal of what has been termed "free anxiety," distributed widely through almost all the patient's thinking. In such a situation as this latter there is not necessarily any immediate or obvious relation between the organic dysfunction and the fear.

I. The first type of case may be described as illness under conditions such that the necessary assurance is almost automatic in the situation. In three continents I have happened across country districts in which the local physician was a first-class medical man practicing there because he liked the life of the countryside and disliked cities or crowded industrial centers. The chief local occupation was farming of various types, the social interrelation of the various family groups was complex and strong. Add to this an immense, and justified, confidence in the competence of the physician and my picture is complete. Even in these days of crowded city life one can discover a few instances of somewhat similar situations; for instance, if a child falls ill of mumps or measles in a well-ordered house in a well-ordered residential district, if a member of an athletic team or a soldier in wartime is injured, there is immediately available a competent physician who is known to the patient.

In instances such as these the need of assurance is in the charge of a closely united social group. The physician is an active member of the group and must know how to identify himself with the social reassurance function as he proceeds to technical examination. But everything in the surrounding is saying to the patient, "Here is the doctor. *Now* you will be all right." Since the patient usually knows the doctor personally and has known him for years, he is also saying this to himself. There is what one might call a total conspiracy of reassurance. Everyone takes the ailment as obvious; no one is frightened. This is almost a social ritual, and is automatic.

II. This almost automatic social assurance was at one time more general than it is now; it may indeed have been universal in the earlier stages of our history. Here may perhaps be found the historic justification of that seeming neglect of medical schools to study the human being as well as the ailment—the neglect of which I spoke earlier. But the physician of these days can no longer assume social collaboration of this extensive and adequate type in his ordinary consultations. The second type of case I specify must therefore be regarded as representing the usual or average medical consultation of today. The patient knows little or nothing of the doctor; he has been "sent" by someone, friend or physician. And the physician knows little or nothing of the patient—his family, his daily work, his social affiliations. In this situation the second diagnosis, the localization of the need of assurance, suddenly becomes more important. Little or no assistance, explicit or implied, can be expected from the patient's immediate and social background. The instances I cite under this general heading develop from the simple to the less simple.

(a) The most simple instance is that in which the assurance needed relates itself directly to the ailment or to a symptom. A patient with abdominal pain, for example, has given much thinking to identification of the pain with gastric ulcer or malignancy. Success in treating the organic disorder depends in part on discovering what the patient is frightened of as a result of "overthinking." An eminent physician, now in retirement, tells himself that in later middle age while still active he noticed that he was becoming breathless after mounting stairs. He reflected uneasily that he should perhaps consult a specialist colleague. Then one day as he came out of the subway he noticed that he was more breathless than usual. Suddenly he remembered that he had ascended on the escalator and had not mounted steps at all. He laughed and lost both the fear and the symptom. The physician being a skilled person could thus reassure himself or, rather, could be directly reassured by the obvious absurdity of the situation. The average patient without technical knowledge requires skilled assistance, and assurance, before he can develop such a point of view.

(b) The next instance cited is a situation in which the assurance demanded may have no direct relevance to the ailment protested. The assurance demanded is nevertheless particular and not necessarily evidence of a general anxiety. An industrial nurse, whose mornings were occupied in the conduct of a small clinic in a factory, made some interesting observations of this type of case. After two years of work in the factory, she came to know a considerable number of workers rather intimately. Being a good interviewer and observer, she noticed that it was rarely the minor casualty, for example, a cut or splinter, that brought a worker to her. Frequently, the worker would dress such an injury himself in a rough manner and without leaving his job. On the mornings that he brought such an injury to her for attention, there was some other matter he wished to discuss. And it was always a problem with respect to which he needed assurance. It might be medical—his own health or that of some member of his family—or it might be social—a son, daughter, or wife. The nurse became very alert to, or it might be said expectant of, the second consultation. A patient may bring a minor ill to a physician when he really wishes to consult him on another problem. This is the more characteristic the better he knows his physician.

(c) The reassurance must be addressed to the appropriate person, who is not always the patient himself. A girl does very well in her studies at college but does not find herself at ease with her associates. She does not go to dances as they do; she does not know any young men. She is apt to feel the social disability most acutely during the general chatter at mealtime; she develops globus hystericus. This does not trouble her greatly until she returns home for the holidays. Her father—sensitive, intelligent, educated—becomes alarmed and takes her to a throat specialist. The specialist sees the girl alone and speedily loses interest; he pushes her off with a vague assurance that she will be all right. He does not see the father except to say farewell. The father, still dissatisfied, goes to his physician. The latter, realizing that assurance is needed, explains the condition at length, and the father finally is comforted. When the father is reassured, the daughter's symptom begins to abate.

Two comments suggest themselves. The first is obvious, namely, that in such a case effective assurance is the most important part of the treatment. Further, the assurance must not be addressed to the patient only but to any person in her immediate social context whose affection and alarm provoke a consequent increase of alarm in her.

The second comment is an observation on the effect of diminished social contacts upon family life. In a small and ordered society the closely organized family operates, like the social group itself, to support the doctor and reassure the patient. In a situation

I

where social contacts are weakened or diminished, the highly organized family operates in a contrary manner. Its isolation reinforces its anxiety; it tends therefore to alarm and to exaggeration of the ill rather than to reassurance.

III. The third type of case includes the really frightened people, those people who suffer a general alarm about themselves, their health, their position in the world. In such cases the ailment may itself be organic only in a minor fashion: it may in a sense be provoked, and it will surely be exaggerated, by the terror and general need of 'assurance. These cases are the exact contrary of the first type: in the first type the social system conspires to reassure; in this third type the lack of assured functional relation to the social system is conspiring to produce a sense of insecurity and terror.

(a) The simplest cases are instances of what Durkheim has called *anomie*.[2] A woman of seventy enters the outpatient department of a hospital complaining of pain in her legs. The hospital records show that she has periodically entered herself with this complaint over a number of years. The medical examiners have tended to refer her to the psychiatrists and the psychiatrists to send her back to the medical clinic. Encouraged to talk, she explained that for most of her life she had been a working housekeeper in hotels

---

[2]Emile Durkheim, *Le Suicide* (Paris: Librarie Felix Alcan, 1897), p. 281.

and successful in that function. Having saved money, she determined to "retire" when the economic depression diminished the amount of such work required. She acquired a room and furnished it; she developed a routine of living. The effect of this newly acquired routine of living was to shut her off from all active or effective human contacts. If she talked to women they "talked only of their troubles"; there was no other person with whom she could talk. It was after some months of this isolation that she presented herself at the hospital. For a person who has been continually active, who is still amazingly serene in the circumstances, this functionless style of living constitutes a major dysfunction. While this aspect of her situation was being made clear, she dropped all reference to and apparently forgot the pain in her legs. The hospital attempted to develop new and satisfactory human relationships for her.

This case relates itself to the experiences, quoted above, of the industrial nurse. It is a more complicated development of the same type of situation. The individual is unable herself to make articulate the nature of the dysfunction; but she is aware of an exaggeration of the organic condition, and her limited capacity for thought and expression lights upon this, the organic condition, for complaint to the physician. The physician naturally is unable to confirm this expression.

(b) A chance phrase dropped inadvertently by a physician may seem in such cases actually to pro-

voke a disorder. This is not suggestion or suggestibility; there is no imitation of the appropriate organic
symptoms as in hysteria. In one of the three well-
ordered country districts of which I spoke above,
the authorities decided to institute a high school. The
newly appointed headmaster came from a large city;
and, some six months after his arrival, he presented
himself in the physician's consulting rooms and asked
for a medical examination. A short conversation
showed that he was not a candidate for life insurance,
that he had suffered no accident, that he complained
of no particular symptoms. The physician found
himself somewhat puzzled by a consultation quite
outside the ordinary run of his practice; however, he
proceeded to subject his patient to an extremely
careful examination. He found nothing that could
be reported as variant from what might be expected
in a normal person of the patient's age, other than a
certain suggestion of apprehension. As the patient
left him, he said more by way of conversation than
diagnosis, "Your heart's a bit sluggish; don't get
influenza." The patient left him, and a week or so
later—in 1918—the alarm of "Spanish Influenza" began. The patient lapsed into a condition of extreme
anxiety and had to be sent to the city for medical
care.

In this instance study of the individual showed
that he had never in any real or human sense "be-
longed" to a group of people. It was this, rather than
any mere city-bred character, which made him so

utterly foreign to the country district. A solitary boyhood with few companions had been followed by an adolescence in which he had worked desperately for distinction in the educational system and had in some measure succeeded. Then an unfortunate incident—while staying in the house of an acquaintance he had seduced a maidservant and had felt it his duty to marry her. His wife was a pleasant, uneducated creature, utterly unfitted to be the comrade of an educator. This fact still further separated him from his fellows, and he became a prey to a heavy conviction of sin and to forebodings of calamity. His foreboding took the form of hypochondriacal alarms about his health. It was these alarms, and his general feeling that he was a social outcast, that took him into the consulting rooms of the physician.

Instances such as this may be multiplied almost indefinitely in any modern industrial or business center. They may seem to approximate or to shade into those cases that demand the special care and attention of the psychiatrist. Nevertheless it must be said that it is not intelligent or sensible for medicine to seek to unload all the personal problems it encounters upon the already overburdened shoulders of the psychiatrist. Furthermore, while many of these cases do not benefit greatly by prolonged "analysis," it is invariably necessary that something should be done to alter and amend effectively their social situation.

At this point I must pause to call attention to an interesting development in the theme of this address. I began by observing that a patient requires of his physician not only medical diagnosis but also personal assurance. I attempted to devise an arbitrary and empirical classification of three types of personal situation—the classification based upon an approximate estimate of the kind of fear an individual suffers and its distribution in his thinking. It is now apparent that observation of the type and extent of assurance needed has become observation also of the kind of social situation in which the patient habitually finds himself, the kind of social conditioning that has produced him. The individual who lives in a small and ordered community requires small assurance; the whole social situation, of which the physician is an essential part, conspires to reassure him. In a larger society an individual assured of his place and function may as a patient require assurance. But in this instance the assurance is probably more or less particular, more or less easily discovered—it is something left over, as it were, by the social order. At the extreme end of the scale is the individual who gets no assurance from this surrounding: on the contrary, his lack of continuous and intimate relationship with others inspires in him a fund of free anxiety, which attaches itself to all he thinks. In brief, one may claim that the need of assurance is an index not only of personal but of social well-being. The large-scale modern society very easily develops patches of social disintegration, of diminished human association. Within such patches is found great human unhappiness, which cannot be explained by the usual economic, psychological, or political studies. This observation has importance not only for medical practice but for every human activity. The administrator in business or industry is already aware of increasing difficulty in the task of securing continuous and wholehearted coöperation from large associations of people. Diminished faith in the society shows itself in medicine as an increased need for assurance: it shows itself in industry as disquiet, unrest, disorder. Diminished social order—frightened people.

In these days it is characteristic that the small, well-ordered society is becoming less common, the large industrial and populous centers more common. Especially in these days then the physician in his ordinary practice must address himself to two diagnoses—the one a diagnosis of the medical ill in the strict sense; the other a diagnosis of the need of assurance. This latter involves careful investigation of the present situation of the individual, and of his personal and social history. It is no doubt possible sometimes to mitigate or banish an organic ill without the second diagnosis: but it is not possible so to *cure* the patient. The patient is not fully cured until he is himself certain of his restoration to health. Confidence in his medical attendant is established when the relevant personal situation has been brought to light. This is evidenced by a sudden disposition in the patient to "unload" everything upon the doctor. The capacity for assurance that a physician develops in such a context is astonishing—unnecessary pains and other symptoms will disappear almost at a word.

The physician who follows such a method has the satisfaction of knowing that he has been of immense aid to a fellow human being. I hope I have made it clear that he has the further satisfaction of knowing that he has contributed some small item of knowledge to the difficult problems—personal, social, political—of our difficult age.

INDEX

Printed and bound by CPI Group (UK) Ltd, Croydon, CR0 4YY

01/11/2024

01782616-0003